Praise for Eat Sh*t and Die

"Clark has taken the rugged path to recovery. Let him be your sensei on a route that can seem eternally uphill and help you find that way thru."
-Scott Jurek, ultramarathon champion, bestselling author of NORTH and Eat and Run

"If you've read David Clark's work or know anything about his life, you know he's introspective, honorable, humble, and open to new ideas. But when he makes a decision, he's a relentless motherfucker. David Clark is my friend. He's hung in my house. We're fathers, sons, and recovering addicts. David's made me laugh and cry. He's always inspiring me. I'm not sure if 'Eat Sh*t and Die' makes me want to hug him or strangle him because it's so on point about me and about what I need to do for myself. I guess if anyone's going to tell me exactly what's going on and how I can make things better for my kids' future, it might as well be my friend, David Clark."
- Tom Arnold, Actor, Comedian, Television Host

"David Clark is one of the most unique individuals I have ever met. The way he can frame and present his complex thoughts in an easy-to-understand way is pure genius. His book kept me up all night long and impacted me very deeply. I recommend it to everyone."

- Stone Cold Steve Austin, action movie icon and WWF Superstar

"David is a beacon of hope to those that struggle with food. In 'Eat Sh*t and Die,' he gives readers exactly what they need to understand that addiction is so much more than indulgence. David has traveled this path, and his experience and advice are invaluable to anyone that is seeking change and hope."

- Tim Kaufman, Author, and Host of FatManRants.Com

"David seems to be in touch with a deeper meaning that translates into all he does. His message of hope and dedication to better yourself is life changing."

- Luc Robitaille, President, Los Angeles Kings, NHL Hall of Fame

"Direct and funny - an absolute lighthouse for those lost and looking for a way to become healthier and happier."

*   - Amy Freeze, ABC New York*

"The book that will turn the weight-loss industry on its ear. Bravo David Clark for having the courage to write 'Eat Sh*t And Die."

*   - Dr. Vassily Eliopoulos, MD*

David Clark

Eat Sh*t And Die:
Radical Rehab for Food Junkies And Sugar Addicts

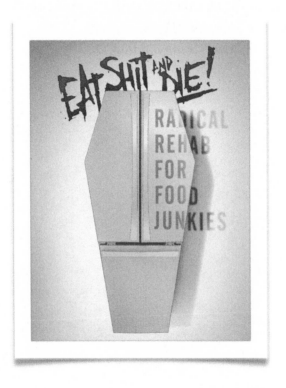

David Clark

David Clark

In memory of my father, Loren Clark.
Your love kept me alive when I forgot how to breathe.
See you on the other side, Warrior.

Foreword

David could not be writing this book at a more critical time. According to the Centers for Disease Control, as of 2018, 42.4% of Americans are obese, which is an astonishing increase from the 30.5% figure we saw in 2000. Notably, this is without considering individuals classified as overweight. Obesity has become an epidemic in the Western world, and it often becomes a life-long struggle. Research suggests that 55% of obese children go on to become obese in adolescence, which 80% of those individuals remaining become obese into young adulthood. So why is this happening?

Based on the United States Department of Agriculture (USDA) food supply data, Americans are eating more sugar, refined grains, meat, and added fats such as oil and butter than ever before! Added fats alone made up 23% of the total caloric intake of Americans as of 2010, while fruit consumption remained unchanged, and vegetable consumption actually dropped by 2% since 1970. Not only are we eating more than ever, but what we are eating is complete junk!

David Clark

I believe the issue lies much deeper than just knowing these foods are not doing us any good. We are drawn to them. Biologically, we want those calorie-rich, sweet, and salty foods, and sometimes our biology can overpower our minds. It's not like anybody truly believes the candy bar or bacon grease are healthy foods, but sometimes we just can't help it. I, too, was a victim of this as a child.

I spent the first 15 years of my life struggling with weight. As a child, I even tried the Atkins diet to no avail. After all, how could anyone expect a child to stay away from the candy cupboard at home or the snacks provided at recess? It wasn't until I fundamentally changed my relationship with food that I was able to overcome the addiction and actually see results. It took something internal for me to make a connection with my health struggles.

Suffering from asthma as a child and having tried just about every diet fad in the hopes of losing weight, I decided to give ditching dairy a try. To my surprise, my asthma vanished. I no longer needed my salbutamol inhaler for PE class or soccer games. For the first time in a long time, I could breathe deep. This was the driver for me adopting, and most importantly, maintaining a healthier diet. It wasn't a short-term fix, but for long-term health.

As you can see, sometimes the science isn't enough. Simply knowing the facts won't get you the results if you've succumbed to the stranglehold of addiction. That's where David's program comes in. While I may not have progressed through the three stages of recovery in the exact format David lays out in this book, I come to the same conclusions and make the same adjustments in my own life to ultimately find long-term success. And by following his program, I'm sure you too can break free from the shackles of food addiction.

Dr. Matthew Nagra, N.D.

Ground Zero

"Life is like a box of chocolates - it won't last very long if you're fat."
- David Clark

"There are two mistakes one can make along the road to truth - not going all the way, and not starting."
– Buddha

Welcome to rehab. You might not know it, but you are at rock bottom. Your life has gotten out of control, and you are afraid of what's going to happen if you don't change. I know this is true because you have taken action. You've taken a step you hope can put an end to the runaway train that your eating has become. We rarely do things on a whim, and a series of emotional events brought you to this moment, so whether you bought this book with an amused smile on your face or shameful tears in your eyes, I am guessing there is a certain amount of pain that brought you here. I know firsthand that it doesn't feel good to be fat.

It doesn't feel good to know you have failed repeatedly to get yourself to do something that you know you should do. Something you *want* to do, in fact. Something that you know will make you a happier and better person. It doesn't feel good to feel weak-minded, gluttonous, or that you are helpless and lost. Yet, you instinctively know the only thing that will break this cycle of depression once and for all is putting an end to your destructive relationship with food. That's why you're here. That's what connects us. Even if you aren't quite there yet, even if you aren't sold on the idea that you are one-hundred percent addicted to food or that your life is out of control, I promise you that this program will open your eyes to how profoundly food affects you.

I hope to expose you to exactly how much of your relationship with eating is an illusion and to introduce you to some practices that will restore health and balance to your life. Let me be clear: the methods, ideas, and concepts in this book have been developed over a decade of working directly with people trying to solve this health-balance riddle. I created this program while helping people lose thousands of pounds, change their daily habits, and become totally new versions of themselves. My program is a blend of Buddhism, athleticism, cynicism, vegetarianism, "heavy-metalism," and a few other "isms" all blended together. That being said, the magic isn't in my program - it's in you. Yes, you will receive everything you need to wholly and radically change your life here, but the information itself will only possess value if you choose to act, if you wish to receive it with a humble and open heart.

I chose to write this book for many reasons, one was money - tons of money, and of course, let's not forget the fame and the adoration of the media. Okay, seriously now. Even if, for some odd reason, those were attainable by writing this book, I know better than to do anything solely for the purpose of making money. It was the relentless pursuit of money and material success that caused me to become painfully lost so many years ago.

By the time I turned twenty-nine years of age, I was living a life that seemed absolutely impossible, given how I grew up. Although my ferocious pursuit of material wealth helped focus me long enough to overcome the weight of a rocky childhood, it did not deliver me the state of happiness and satisfaction I was led to believe it would. After spending most of my childhood living in campgrounds, church parking lots, and shelters, I settled down in Colorado, grabbed a GED, wormed my way into college, took a part-time job selling mattresses, and ended up owning a chain of thirteen retail furniture stores earning over eight million dollars a year - not bad for a kid that used to fish aluminum cans out of dumpsters to bring home a couple of bucks for groceries.

Yet, the houses, cars, and expanding bank account didn't do anything to fill the hole in my broken heart. By the time I hit thirty-four, I had weighed three-hundred-twenty pounds, I was bankrupt, I had a heart condition and disastrously high blood pressure. I was also drinking two bottles of scotch a day, I was abusing prescription medication, and I was wearing out the road between my house and the McDonald's on the street corner.

I was committing suicide in the worst possible way anyone could - slowly, every day, on the thirty-year plan. But I didn't die, and that's the point - I did what I have heard people say over and over again is impossible - I changed. Not just my weight, but who I was. The person writing this book in no way resembles that bloated drunk from my past. The mirror no longer recognizes the look of confusion, desperation, and defeat I brought to it every day for decades. Today it knows a different chap, one that offers up a healthy, fit, and athletic body every morning. A reflection that projects a confident smile that has over fourteen years of sobriety pulling up at the corners. A man that rises with the sun, has an energetic zest for life, peaceful nature, and the ability to remain calm in a world of chaos.

But who cares about *MY* journey? I am sure you aren't reading this because you want to know that I was able to turn *MY* life around, but more likely because you have a journey of your own you'd like to take - a change you'd like to make for yourself. I'm reasonably sure that one of the things you want to change is that pesky, arrogant son of a bitch three-digit number that appears on the scale every morning when you stand on it. That is the real reason I wrote this book. Because I know from the bottom of my heart that I am not a special case. I didn't game the system, or beat the odds, although many will tell you I did just that. I just followed a path to real change. That path is there for any person that wants to become new.

In my experience, people don't fail to lose weight and keep it off because they aren't strong enough, or because they don't have enough will power. They fail for very specific and very avoidable reasons that we will go into at great length. But the essence of the message here is simple - you CAN do this. As sure as you are reading these words, you can make this the very last time that you ever have to start again - I promise you that. I have run some of the world's toughest races, I have set records as an athlete, I have written two bestselling books, and I coach athletes all over the world. Yet, I am the same guy that used to lay on the floor crying because I couldn't get myself to follow through on anything. If that isn't solid proof that everyone can change who they are - I don't know what is.

Let me be very clear: This is not a scientific weight-loss study or technical manual on nutrition. I am not going to throw mindless data at you in an effort to show you how everyone in the industry has it wrong, and how I have it right. I won't be droning on through the book about what our ancestors ate, what people will eat in the future, what celebrities know and aren't telling you, or anything about which clinics have released previously unknown nutritional secrets. What I will be spending most of my time talking about *you*. I hate to be the one that breaks it to you, but you know the real problem that needs to be addressed here, right? The Big Kahuna in the mirror - you and maybe more accurately - how you see yourself.

Before you get the wrong impression, this isn't one of those trendy "tough love" types of books where I call you a "pussy" and tell you to "cowboy up," although I may say things like that from time to time. This book is about the truth. Sometimes the truth is harsh, hard to hear, and painful, but I won't be going after you just for shock value. But this is a not philosophy book either. I am not going to attempt to construct a deep ethereal argument that shows how society has failed us, how our weight issues fit into a greater human problem, or how you need only to change your mind to change your habits. This is a book with an agenda, a timeline, and an action plan. I want you to take actions that will immediately impact how you think, what you do, and who you are. You won't have to wonder how to apply the concepts I sketch out here; I am going to map out a ten-step path to freedom that will allow you to throw that old self-destructive "you" under the bus and then back over it a few times to make sure it's dead.

You've probably heard of "The Four Agreements," and if you haven't, you should look up the book. If you do, you will find four simple truths that, if you put into practice, will help you experience a happier and less stressful life. Well, my book is more like *The Four Fucks*. The food addicts guide, written by a former fat person, addressing why you are fucked, how you got fucked, who is doing the fucking, and how the fuck you can change it. I do this because I respect you enough to give you the truth. I'm not going to pump you up with a bunch of feel-good inspiration and send you into the world to get your face kicked in. I will tell you directly what I know to be real, and it will always come from a place of love. If the words are uplifting and motivational -

David Clark

great. If they scare you or piss you off - so be it. Either way, we will be in this together each step of the way. I believe the most courageous act that any human will ever undertake is the willingness to look at themselves honestly, accept the reality of where they are, and then make improvements. That is precisely what brought us together today.

My suggestion is to read this book in its entirety before starting the program. There will be broad concepts and ideas explained in detail at the beginning, and then the concepts will be more specifically integrated into the ten-step **Radical Rehab** program. The "guts" of the program is broken into a "Prehab" and "Three Stages." In the Prehab, I address the reasons and causes for why so many suffer from food addiction and obesity.

The plan itself is broken into three separate stages. Stage 1 focuses on getting your house in order. Stage 2 focuses on your mind and spirit, and Stage 3 focuses on changing your body. It should be clear to you that each step builds on the previous. So in essence, we will be placing a pot on the stove, and with each new stage we will be adding to the recipe as we go, never taking anything out of the pot, but always adding more new concepts and practices until at the end we have completed a "new life soup" ready for consumption. At the very end of the book, I will put it all together for you in a concept you can follow to free yourself and live the life you deserve – happy, healthy, and no longer eating yourself to death.

PREHAB

Chapter 1
Why Are We Fat?

"My good health is my outer wealth."
— *Sri Chinmoy*

Today, half of our entire country is overweight, and almost forty percent of us are obese. Even in the state I live in, Colorado, which has been voted one of the healthiest places in the United States, I still see obese people everywhere. Yeah, it's true, I also see a lot of "26.2" and "Ironman" bumper stickers, but that's still a small fraction of the state's population. It seems like McDonald's and The Bachelor have a lot in common. When asked, everyone says they don't get it, but yet somehow, over a billion burgers are sold every year.

The reason why people are so overweight is junk food works. It does the intended job. The problem is the job performed doesn't match the description of the job that needs to be done. Food is meant to supply us energy, sustenance, and the raw materials to keep the human-machine working. But instead, without even realizing it, we have bestowed on food the job of making us feel good. Sure, it enters the picture through a more evolutionary introduction - hunger.

David Clark

But once the hunger arrives, we use our less informed base instincts to seek out "what sounds good," not what will sustain us and keep us healthy. When we eat foods high in fat, salt, and sugar, it *feels* good while we are eating it, even if it means our bodies are left starving for the micronutrients needed to be healthy. There wouldn't be a fast-food restaurant on every corner of the world if it weren't meeting the expectations of its customers. But that begs a very important question: What are our expectations when it comes to food? Certainly, if we expected to be nourished, energized, and invigorated by our trip to the burger store, then we would discontinue our daily trips to said establishment. But we aren't asking that of our food, and that is a very big part of the problem.

Most of the time, civilized humans pride themselves on acting intelligently and being completely rational. Humans wouldn't choose to take a longer route to work, knowing they would arrive late. Instead, they factor in the various route options, calculate traffic patterns, past experiences, and choose what is deemed to be the best-calculated option. It is done knowing that it may end up being an incorrect assessment, but nevertheless, it deserves consideration.

We as humans negotiate the price of cars, houses, our salaries, etc., and we do so because no one wants to make poor choices that will come back to haunt them. Yet, we completely abandon our previously esteemed analytical commitment when it comes to food because we are blinded by the immediate feeling of pleasure that comes from shoving fat and sugar into our mouths.

Many times, we know the foods we are eating are unhealthy. We aren't completely delusional enough to think a Big Mac will improve our health. Astonishingly, we openly accept that after eating our junk food lunch, we will feel lethargic, slow, and most likely guilty. Yet we willingly operate under the self-prescribed illusion that we will get some greater benefit from eating the food than the certain boomerang after-effect. Although we repeat this pattern over and over, each time we find a way to ignore all previous experiences and jump back on the junk food carousel. So why do we self-destruct like this, you ask? Why do we even crave this food if it's poison? Let's go deeper…

The reason for this perpetual junk food cycle is *not* because we are somehow predisposed to double cheeseburgers or cheesecake, as we are led to believe. The environment in which humans evolved into the most efficient, powerful, and magical machines in the cosmos didn't include these toxic combinations. We are unwitting victims to the most elegant guiding system ever made - survival instinct. Our bodies instinctively know what they need to repair, to thrive, and to move. When our electrolyte balance is off, we crave salty things. When we need highly biochemical food for neurological function, we crave fats like avocados and nuts. When our blood sugar is low, we crave sugary things like strawberries and oranges. But we evolved these cravings in a time of caloric

David Clark

scarcity. Just surviving a single day was a successful experience for our prehistoric ancestors. In the Paleolithic era, humans with the instinct and preference for salty, sugary, highly fatty, and calorically dense foods naturally survived better than their Epicurious neighbors.

Most early humans died of starvation, not by "dinosaur bite," as we may envision. In other words, you and I arrived here on millions of years of adaption fueled by the intense desire for fat and sugar, yet our cravings evolved outside the world of modern processed food. So, when your Cro-Magnon brain turns up a sugar craving to fix a drop in energy levels, and you give it a Pepsi instead of a handful of berries, it goes into euphoria-pleasure-processing overload. In an instant, any thoughts of grapes or melons have been cast aside in favor of the refined sugar. With this previously unknown chemical ingested, the body requires very little work on a cellular level to convert calories to glucose or even to break it down for digestion - the processed corn syrup simply "jumps" right into the bloodstream. The problem is this happens at a high cost physically and psychologically. You are overwriting millions of years of programming by giving the body a food-related experience so deeply pleasurable that the brain places this new behavior at the top of the priority list. The brain is still operating under the old laws of scarcity when it does this, so it sees no potential danger in rewarding behavior that will keep it alive - which of course, is its ultimate goal.

After years of abuse by these engineered food-substances, the body isn't even mildly interested in the natural foods that will deliver it more sustainable, long-term energy. Instead, it wants a quick fix. As a result, you get caught in a pleasure loop that eventually becomes the default program for making all food choices. The biological evolutionary instincts that once saved your ancestors are now working against you. Your cravings are currently taking place outside of the rational decision-making part of your brain, so you aren't even aware of the undesired effect of these poisonous man-made foods.

This is the same cycle that can make addicts out of prescription painkiller users. A patient might start with an opioid prescription for a broken arm, but behind the scenes, undiagnosed emotional pain may also be served. The bone eventually heals, but the body is still craving the opiate, based on its ancillary rewards. The prescription runs out, the withdrawal kicks in, and next thing you know, the addict is on the streets trying to buy more. Only, in a food-induced addiction cycle, you aren't heading to the proverbial skid-row of losing your job, your house, and your marriage; instead you are slowly devolving into a ravished metabolic wasteland. Until one day, you can scarcely use your fat for energy. Your body, designed by millions of years of biological evolution to be a fat-burning machine, has become a fat-storing machine, and you struggle to just to move about the day. Always feeling sluggish, worn out, and tired, using refined sugar in the form of coffee, donuts, and energy-drinks to crawl from feeding to feeding. It's not just our energy levels that suffer. When the body isn't working well, all its functions retard - our cognitive ability, our emotional patterns, and even our mental health.

So, what does this all mean? It means our bodies are programmed using evolutionary code, not the language of today's comfort food. If cavemen would have had access to grocery stores and fast-food restaurants, it is very likely that you and I would not be here, and the humans that *would* be here would have a whole new set of adaptations. Maybe ones that included the ability to live off simple sugars without becoming diabetic, or the ability to eat animal fat without accumulating cholesterol, clogged arteries, and cancer. Or maybe these new humans would have evolved because of a mutation that gave them a desire for healthy foods that would make them live longer, be more active, more healthy, and appear more desirous as mates - now that makes more sense to me.

It's more likely in these imaginary early days of humans, the fast-food junkies would have died off and never made it - too slow to avoid prey, too bloated and unhealthy to attract mates, and not around long enough to produce viable offspring. Kind of makes you wonder where we are heading now, huh? Woah... wait a minute. Did I just say skinnier people are more desirous as mates? Yeah, I did... sort of. But only in the sense that sexual attraction comes from a deep desire to attract what we perceive as a healthy mate that will produce healthy offspring. I am pretty sure at three-hundred-twenty pounds and choking down my twentieth barbecue chicken wing, no one would have mistaken me for a healthy choice for a mate. Keep in mind, I am talking only in terms of biological evolution. I am aware that we are no longer in a world where only base desires rule behavior.

As large food companies have materialized, and "food engineering" has become an industry, millions of products have been created to meet the demand for sugary and highly fatty foods. It wasn't even until the turn of the century that we ate anything that wasn't a "whole food," and since then, the lines between pleasure delivery and nourishment become more and more blurred. Just as modern medicine has exacerbated the opiate addiction crisis by developing more potent and stronger pain medications that elevate both physical and emotional pain, the tendency for "food-abuse" has also become closer and closer to the norm. This is because food wasn't intended to be a mechanism for handling stress, escaping pain, dealing with loss, or feeling pleasure. I am not saying eating shouldn't be a pleasurable experience; certainly it should be just that, but it shouldn't be the sole purpose of eating - and if you turn on the television, it's not hard to see we are obsessed with food nowadays.

The larger the role *food obsession* factors into our lives, the more we regress in the ability to simply handle the ups and downs of life while just sitting still with our mouths closed. When I look back at my own relationship to food, it occurred to me that I lived

David Clark

most of my life as if I was my own dog - always rewarding myself for good behavior with a treat always equating food with love. But we are not dogs. Dogs could teach us much about how to be happy and present in the moment after dinner time is over.

At the risk of sounding like the Boulder hippie most people think I am, I do believe many of the problems that face us as a society can be traced back to our relationship with food. Meaning we are increasingly disconnected from ourselves and from each other. Our entire days have become one giant mashup of never-ending activity from the time we wake until the time we go to bed. Our minds are capable of accomplishing anything if we give it a singular focus, yet we cannot even separate our morning coffee, from checking emails, and paying bills. We go instantly from the shower, to the breakfast table, driving to work, executing our daily duties, and coming home as if it were one giant activity. One constant bombardment of images and conversations into the consciousness until eventually, we have so many windows opened on our human-computer, that a simple thought sends the pinwheel turning and turning unable to download anything new.

We have lost the ability to simply "be." We don't sit and enjoy a cup of coffee for the wonderful experience it is. We don't fall in love with the act of driving our cars. We don't separate the things we do into individual experiences, and as a result, our brains never shut down. We can scarcely sit without being overrun by all the thoughts that we keep in a perpetual spin cycle. In response, many of us have learned to eat to try to break the cycle. We eat when we're bored, and we eat when we're busy. We eat when we're happy and when we're sad. We eat because it creates a few seconds of comfort that overrides all the endless internal chatter. If I had to place my finger on the single biggest reason most people are unable to moderate what they eat, it comes down to one missing thing - patience. Axl Rose was right, "All we need is just a little patience." This book, in part, is about teaching you the patience needed to do all the things you have ever wanted to do.

We will work on the spiritual stuff and how mindfulness plays a role in our health later. For now, let's get back to why we are so fat. It may come as a shock to some of you, but obesity is as much about malnourishment as it is overeating. I *will* say it's *more* about malnourishment. It's easy to think of obesity as a condition brought on by gluttony, and there *was* a time in history when that was accurate but gone are the days of such a simple dichotomy. Today's processed foods have an underestimated impact on how the body converts energy, repairs muscle, triggers hunger, and stores fat. There was a time when almost everything that a person might eat throughout the day was a *real food.* Meaning a real, whole food as nature intended it to work in our specifically evolved biology. Simple - you got hungry; you ate. Your body would use the calories to fuel various metabolic and biological functions, and when you "ran out," you would get hungry again. If you did a lot of work that day, your appetite was large, if you were not as active… you get the point.

For a person to grow obese under this scenario, they would need to eat past the normal rise and fall of appetite. They would have to eat even in the absence of hunger, and it would be very gluttonous by definition. Not surprisingly, the hand of natural selection created a human animal with a homeostatic environment where hunger and appetite were reasonably balanced. It's worth noting that until the advent of the modern human, no animal has ever had to "portion control," they simply ate when hungry. It wasn't until we started domesticating animals and feeding them our processed foods that we started to see things like obese pets and animal diabetes. Think about that…

Today's processed foods have been, for lack of a better description, "chemically digested" before they make it to our stomachs. The procedure for creating a processed food includes breaking down a formally whole food into base components and reassembling them in a packaged form that it can be preserved in so they can sit on shelves without rotting. This takes all the work out of the digestion process for our bodies. As these manufactured foods land in the acid-vat of our stomachs, the chemically altered substance immediately disintegrates before digestion even begins. As a result, the calories, now in the form of carbs, fat, and protein, are rapidly absorbed into our bloodstream. This circumvents hours of slow-digesting, elevated metabolic function, and balanced blood sugar levels.

It usually takes hours for the body to process a whole-food, but a cookie can make it through the security line and board the blood-sugar plane in about five minutes - *HIJACKED*! The response to this chemical bomb is an immediate rise in blood sugar as the energy from the engineered food hits the bloodstream all at once. As the flood gates open, the sugar (now in the form of glucose) hits our brain, and we experience an immediate pleasure response as the body senses this new intense energy supply - and *that's* the good news. The bad news is this is just an illusion. There is nothing sustainable in this spike of energy, and the body struggles as the sugar rush quickly dies off.

Just as the blood-sugar spiked in response to the immediate glucose increase, the endocrine system, in fear that the spike was caused by something threatening (like eating of an entire bucket of strawberries), causes the pancreas to secrete insulin into the bloodstream. Insulin is our only internal means to drop blood-sugar back to normal. But there lies an additional problem - you didn't actually *eat* a bucket of strawberries. You only ate a twenty-five-calorie sugar cookie, but because it was absorbed so rapidly into the bloodstream, your body overreacted. Now, here's the real son-of-a-bitch, the insulin doesn't just drop the blood sugar to *normal* - it inadvertently drops it *below* normal level as the short energy supply starts to wear off even before the insulin takes effect. The outcome is you are left with blood-sugar levels now greatly diminished and *lower* than before you ate that little cookie. Guess what mechanism your body uses to increase blood-sugar? The only one it has - it turns on appetite - yes, you get hungry.

This is the never-ending loop that causes people to overeat. Anyone who has sat on the sofa and eaten an entire bag of potato chips while watching television knows this feeling. You are eating, your belly is full, yet the hunger keeps turning on and on and on. If you doubt it is the processed nature of your food, causing this phenomenon, simply try to duplicate this cycle using any whole food. Let's see how many apples or bananas you can eat while watching Netflix for five hours.

Further complicating things is the inexplicable and relatively unexplored nature of what happens at a *cellular* level to trigger appetite in our brains. This is the area that modern science knows the least about and where we need much research. Unfortunately, this is the part we rarely hear about on fitness shows or in Instagram videos about weight-loss. We think of food in the macronutrient sense - carbs, fats, and proteins. But the micronutrients have more of a role in hunger than we may be willing to accept. Just as the body "turns on" hunger to raise falling blood sugar levels, the body turns on hunger when we are missing essential micronutrients such as vitamins and minerals.

We need micronutrients to repair cellar structures and to supply chemical reactions for billions of cells, and if our diets consist mostly of burgers, pizza, and the occasional salad, chances are you are starving to death while living with an overabundance of calories. This is why I feel malnourishment is at the heart of what is making us fat. It's not that we are simply weak-minded or gluttonous. If we fuel our bodies with the micro building blocks it needs, we will experience robust and efficient chemical reactions, better emotional stability, and the cessation of chronic appetite warfare. We'd also get a body that is working as intended, not just surviving day to day, meal to meal until disease takes it over.

Many times, we aren't even aware of how poorly our bodies are functioning because we have nothing solid to compare it to. Meaning, you wake up every day, you manage to get to work, and you even feel good enough on occasion to go for a hike or to play basketball... how bad can it be? But it's sort of like you have been driving an old junk car that only has one cylinder firing. Yeah, it's getting you to the store and back, but how long will it last while it's leaking oil and the wheels are falling off? What would it feel like if one day you got into that car and it was finely tuned, all cylinders firing, tires pumped up, and the engine was springing to life under your foot on the gas pedal?

While all this complicated chemically driven chaos is going on in our bodies, our minds are getting hammered by the fitness industry and its marketing leeches selling the "secrets" and latest breakthroughs on how to lose weight. We try something new because it touches our deep desire to be healthy and fit, and it works… for a while. Then we end up fatter, more confused, and more depressed. So, we join another gym or hire another personal trainer who really has no fucking clue what it's like to struggle with the depression that comes from feeling hopelessly fat. Shit, the trainer might even deliver results for a while too, until we stop working out, start wishing for the death of said trainer, and get fed up that the scale number isn't dropping as fast as our checking account balance is.

But in reality, what is truly holding us back is not our workout program, but the long-term chronic metabolic damage caused by our food choices. I don't mean calories; I mean the collateral metabolic failure that has caused you to become a fat-storing machine. I wish it were as simple as "eat Keto" or "only eat from 10 am to 6 pm" or my favorite, "eat less, move more," but it isn't. As a gym owner, I have seen firsthand many overweight people who workout harder and more often than the vast majority of folks. Yet, they get no results. So, let's get real about getting our arms around this problem. Don't fear, because all of this is fixable. You *are* bound by the laws of physics and biology and every human *can* lose weight - permanently. It isn't as hard as you think - it's harder… oops. I know that's a frightening thought, but in a weird way, that's what's going to make it fun.

My guess is in your search to obtain a skinny-jean membership card, you have looked under every rock, bought many pieces of workout equipment and weight-loss books, watched every television show and listened to countless gym salespeople, all with the hope of finding the intuitive or easy way to get healthy. Yet you are still here, still looking. If you haven't realized it yet, I'm not here to sell you a new "easy way"-because there isn't one.

This shit is hard. As someone who is both in recovery from alcohol addiction *and* has achieved long-term weight-loss, I can tell you that weight-loss is way fucking harder than sobriety. There are millions of people in recovery - you can't leave your house without bumping into a sober person. But how many people do you personally know that has lost fifty or one-hundred pounds or more and *kept* it off? But here is the good news, friend. I'm going to show you how to be strong enough to do it the hard way - the way that makes it permanent. I'm not going to help you lose weight. I'm going to help you become stronger than you have ever imagined you could be.

But to come along on this ride, you have to make a simple yet counterintuitive commitment moving forward - you must turn the reins over to me. You have to do something you probably don't do very often - you have to blindly trust that someone else knows more about you than you do. That's fucking brutal - I know, I have been there. But for this to work, you have to accept that maybe I know what I am talking about, and more importantly, that maybe you *don't know* what *you're* talking about. What do you have to lose anyway? Besides all that fat? Hell, you can tell me I'm full of shit at the end, but for now - just crank up the Pantera and bang your head along.

We haven't even touched on the true keys to the kingdom yet, the true North Star that will lead you to everything you want. What is that you ask? Have you ever asked yourself *why* you want to lose weight in the first place? I promise it is not as simple as just wanting to look and feel better. It's deeper. I'll give you a nudge - why do we pursue any of the things we do, even the bad ones? I'll tell you why - because every action we take comes with the hidden hope that it will somehow make us happy. The road to lasting change *is* the road to happiness. If you make happiness your means of travel, everything else you desire will come for the ride.

Chapter 2
Am I Addicted?

"Ice cream is exquisite. What a pity it isn't illegal."
— *Voltaire*

"By sweetening with sugar, we can give a false palatableness to even the most indigestible rubbish."
— *An essay in The New York Times, from 1884*

Before we start our rehab, there is something I need you to know, something that might actually come as a shock. There is no such thing as food addiction… Do I have your attention? Good. Now, relax. If you are like me, you have probably dedicated many hours to wondering if you are in fact, addicted to food. That would make sense, wouldn't it? It might explain why you eat recklessly even when you don't necessarily want to eat at all. It might explain why you eat when you're bored, when you're happy, when you're angry, you're sad, or just watching television. It might explain why it is so difficult for you to regulate your food intake, why you make promises to lose weight only to absentmindedly eat a cookie as if you hadn't just spent an hour thinking about how great to would be to fit into that swimsuit this summer. It could be the reason as to why you aren't always honest about what you eat, to yourself or possibly even to others, and why you sometimes feel guilty after you indulge. I can say that all of those behaviors, *all* of them, are present in every addict.

When I was in the absolute throes of denial with my own food and chemical addictions, I had a thought that turned my world upside down. "I'll bet people that aren't alcoholics don't stay awake at night wondering if they are alcoholics." Damn… Just like that, I realized I was on a collision course that would either run me into the cemetery or into sobriety. But, didn't I just say there was no such thing as food addiction? Yes, I did - and I meant it.

Let me explain. Of course, *addiction* itself is a real thing. A real dark, complicated, and very convoluted thing. If you are struggling with the emotions and cycles I outlined above, then you are likely addicted. The distinction is it isn't *FOOD* you are addicted to. You are addicted to chemically processed, commercially packaged, nutrient-deficient shitstorms that, for some unknown reason, we have collectively chosen to give sanctuary under the label "food." So, the problem isn't really *food* addiction - the problem is what we define as food. Or more succinctly, the problem is what we are addicted to isn't food at all.

So, what is food? We touched on this briefly in the last chapter, but let's go deeper. We can define food as any nutritious substance that people or animals eat or drink, or that plants absorb, in order to maintain life. That works well according to Webster, but in the real world, it isn't nearly as straightforward as that. Because although many of the things we eat today are meeting that minimum standard, they are at the same time lopping years of our lives on the back end. Yes, you can sustain life on Twinkies and bacon grease, but you won't last very long doing it. So, what does that mean, you ask? It means your definition of "food" needs to change if you want your pants size to do the same.

You can't make it a day without hearing something about the epidemic of obesity, or how Americans are addicted to fast-food, but these statements miss the mark entirely. The health problems we face in this country such as obesity, diabetes, heart disease, and a whole host of others are merely the side effects of a much bigger problem - that we have perverted and bastardized our definition of food to the point where almost anything we can shove into our mouths qualifies as such. When we walk down the never-ending aisles at the grocery store, we see what we recognize as food everywhere. Some foods we label as "junk" or "unhealthy," but the point is we consider it all to be food. Until we change our own understanding of what food is, until we narrow the definition to exclude certain groups of edible compounds, we are doomed to bounce up and down, back and forth on a perpetually shifting base of poisonous calories that will always produce the same shaky, flabby, and hollowed structure we call our bodies.

When we choose to open our eyes and see things outside our default perspective, we will, by definition, always see something new - food is no different. But it is a challenging thing to do, to say the least. We don't want to let go of our food treasure chest because baked into our old paradigms (pardon the pun) are all the foods that we have attached comfort, love, and expansive emotional experience. In case the panic is rising in you, I am not suggesting that you have to give up anything you have eaten in the past, forever. But I *am* saying that you must learn to see those things differently if you hope to achieve long-lasting health and weight-loss.

This business of breaking the addiction cycle requires massive effort to make the switch. It requires us to be able to intimately touch our deepest pain to be able to walk away permanently. I want you to take note that this redefining of food is perhaps the biggest roadblock you will face. So, you now are at a fork in the road, on the verge of a new reality. Just like Neo sitting in the chair across from Morpheus, you need to choose whether you take the blue pill or the red pill. You can close this book now, go back to your old life, follow some other diet plan, and never have to challenge yourself on what food is. Or you can take the red pill, complete this **Radical Rehab**, and wake up in a new world where you can experience a better and more authentic life. I am not saying I am the Oracle here, by the way. I don't own the ability to see the future or know the correct path for all to follow. But this program is the only way I know how to make a real change. In my experience, you will *never* change your body by changing your food intake or your habits; you must change how you think so that your old ideas and habits become obsolete.

Years ago, while waiting to board a plane, I noticed a commercial on the monitor that showed a taco that utilized a fried egg as the shell. Just as I was about to comment on how absolutely disgusting that is, the person next to me said, "Oh wow, that looks good, doesn't it?" NO, it didn't... I thought in revulsion. But it did get me thinking. Did that *Franken-taco* really look good to that person? Did it *really* look appetizing? It reminded me of how I used to talk about alcohol in my previous life. I would always say things like, "You know what sounds really good right now? A beer." Even though a beer did sound good, mostly what I was thinking about was thirty beers. I was thinking about getting drunk. I wasn't completely lucid about my desire to inebriate myself, but I wasn't exactly unaware either. It was something in between. Almost as if I was allowing myself the illusion that a beer would be refreshing knowing damn well what would happen after I had one.

I immediately applied that same thought chain to how I interacted with food in my past life, and once again, the template fit. I would think, bacon double cheeseburger, and say, "Oh, that sounds heavenly." But the truth was, it didn't always sound good. There were times when certain foods weren't appetizing at all, yet I would eat them anyway. I'd indulge because I knew when the warm salty fat touched my mouth, and my taste buds sprang to life, I would receive

David Clark

pleasure. It was oddly like sex; you don't always have to be in the mood to know it will feel good once you get going. So, when I got down to it, these cravings or knee jerk responses to junk food were less about how good it sounded and more about how it would make me feel while eating it. Bingo. Now we are on to something.

Most of today's foods seem to be based on some sort of a dare or bet. Who can make the most decadent or deadly combination of sugar and animal fat? We have bacon ice cream, deep-fried Oreos, and pizza with fried chicken as the crust. Now I ask you, does any of that honestly sound good to anyone? Stay with me… try to separate your reaction from the reality. I would submit that it might not sound good from a purely dining perspective. There is little chance that those combinations of food sound good to our actual taste buds. But instead, we layer an internal representation of how awesome it would *feel* as we ate it, over the *anticipation* of how it will taste. Because our food supply has become so toxic, our relationship with eating for health has become equally deformed. The result has been an unhealthy relationship with how food makes us feel. That isn't quite right. When the focus is on the broader perspective, it might be more accurate to say the relationship is about how what we eat makes us *stop* feeling.

As food products have become more about pleasure delivery, they have become less about providing our bodies with what we need to feel good in a *sustainable* way. The tube from your mouth to your ass has become just another revenue stream for those selling something to help deal with the emotional pain of life. We have been mind-fucked into believing that eating is a great way to reward ourselves, change how we feel, or even to express love. Chocolates for your Valentine, cake for mom's birthday, ice cream for when you're sick… Jesus. Then we wonder why we can't convince ourselves to eat an apple when we are hungry? Well, it's because an apple can make you feel amazing an hour after you eat it, but it won't help you when your boyfriend is cheating on you. So, what do we do?

We break the cycle by becoming aware of it, by observing it as it happens and taking note of what a shitty bargain eating for comfort is. Eating to make ourselves happy simply does not work. It gives us a temporary state of joy that is gone almost immediately, leaving in its wake too many health complications to list. If we hope to break this cycle and restore ourselves to a sane and healthy relationship with food, we must become mindful of how food (specifically processed food) traps us in its web.

Keep in mind when we are talking about the emotional effects of eating, it is eating *processed foods,* specifically, that is the problem. All bets are off when you are eating whole foods. If you haven't noticed, there aren't a lot of people addicted to apples. I've never seen anyone eat an entire bucket of broccoli or oranges because they were depressed. It's when we short-circuit the body's *natural* food processing state that we get caught in the addictive and emotional storm of comfort eating. Of all the offenders, including processed fats, processed animal and dairy products, baked goods, and the like, let's be clear - sugar is the devil.

Your body creates very little distinction between refined sugar and opioids, and I am not even joking. Sugar meets all the physiological and behavioral qualifications of being a narcotic - euphoria, crash, withdrawal, and craving - and many studies show that refined sugar has the absolute same effect on your brain as cocaine. Think about that for a second. Now, try to remember the last time you went without having *any* sugar for a while. Have you ever gone a month without sugar? If so, what happened when you returned to it? If you are like most other people and me, you probably had difficulty regulating it. I wouldn't be surprised to hear you woke up the next day with your hand in a five-pound M&M bag, Twizzlers hanging from your butt, and powdered sugar around your mouth. If so, I'm not judging.

When Coca-Cola (currently the single most recognized product in the world) first introduced its product, it had three basic ingredients - the cola nut (a natural source of caffeine), cocaine, and of course, sugar to take away the bitter taste of the concoction. Not surprisingly, the product was an instant success. But here is the part that no one suspected. When eventually Coca-Cola was forced to take the cocaine out of the formulation - it was no less addictive.

People still could not get enough of it… Still think sugar is just an innocent little additive to make things taste better? I suspect people would eat dog shit if there were enough sugar in it.

The sugar industry (and yes, there actually is a sugar industry) has also engaged in many of the evil and devious practices that "Big Tobacco" has been proven guilty of. If you want to really open your eyes to the unimaginable disaster that sugar is, read *A Case Against Sugar* by Gary Taubes, or watch the documentary *Sugar Coated*. You'll learn the history of when sugar first started to appear in food products. You'll learn when the addictive effects of sugar became known; it was a game-changer. Sugar hit the scene in an absolute "Blitzkrieg" way by traders and merchants to get it everywhere in the food supply. Like drug dealers fighting for street corners, food manufacturers competed to find new and inventive ways to transform food products into sugar delivery opportunities.

In the seventies and eighties, the medical field became very concerned about the nations' sugar intake. But just like tobacco, the Sugar Council paid many doctors to endorse sugar as harmless. They then set off on a national campaign to set America's mind at rest that sugar is "just as healthy for you like a glass of milk" (which is ironically true, by the way). Doctors on the payroll of large corporate interests started to appear on news programs every night, stating that it was a medical fact that a bowl of fortified sugary cereal was just as healthy for

David Clark

breakfast like fruit and toast. The same doctors postulated it was a diet in excess of *calories* that caused diabetes, regardless of where those calories came from. This, of course, resulted in the creation of an entire billion-dollar diet-food industry based on reduced-calorie foods.

But we now know that those "doctors" were lying. They were not wrong. They knew sugar was wreaking metabolic havoc on people. They were just bought and paid for, much like the doctors who said smoking cigarettes was a harmless way to relax. So, it really isn't hard to see how we ended up where we are today. The reason there is added sugar in everything from soups, to condiments, to pickles, is because it creates loyal users. If there is sugar in a product, the likelihood that it will be purchased a second, third, fourth time is guaranteed. The other day, I walked into a grocery store with my eleven-year-old daughter, and a very nice lady was standing in the bakery handing out free cookies. The cynical part of me wondered if she learned this from the drug dealers, or if it was the other way around.

Now that I have your heart rate around one-eighty, let me say that I'm not saying you can never have sugar... Better? But I am saying that you should not have *any* sugar while you are trying to lose weight - sorry. You must detox. You must learn to see sugar for the powerful narcotic that it is, so you can learn to respect it. That means understanding that refined sugar has a profound effect on your biochemistry, neurochemistry, and on your emotions as well.

Let's focus for a moment on some sugar math. We know sugar is an easy energy source that disrupts our natural fat-burning operations. We already talked about how in the absence of unnatural options (like sugar), our bodies will construct its own biological metabolic pathways to create energy (fat burning). I'm assuming you wouldn't mind increased calorie burning, higher and more sustainable energy levels, and living off your stored fat, right? So, it's important to understand that when you are trying to re-establish these dormant fat-burning pathways, there is an exponential factor in the equation. Meaning the longer your body goes without sugar, the stronger and more powerful these fat-burning pathways become, until one day, fat burning becomes the preferred path for your body to supply energy.

But I have some tough news for you. One weak moment will send you right back to the starting line. I need to drive that point home - your body will *not* make the complete switch over to efficient and long-term fat burning with *any* amount of sugar present in your body, even if sugar only makes a brief appearance, the whole thing collapses, and you have to start again from the beginning. I estimate that ninety-nine out of one-hundred people that try to kick the sugar habit fail for one reason - they don't go long enough to detox. You have to achieve complete sugar sobriety while you are losing weight. But the good news is after you make this biologic adaptation, you can, in theory, have sugar again if you choose to do so, but only in small amounts. However, inviting

David Clark

sugar back into your home is a slippery slope and could send you back to rock bottom... more on that later.

There is also a neurological relationship with your eating practices. Just as your metabolism will take its foot off the gas when simple sugars appear, your brain also struggles with regulating emotions when highly euphoric foods enter the bloodstream. If you get an immediate, and impactful high from that Mountain Dew, your brain makes the association that a simple craving results in an immediate reward. That's a much more direct route from "A" to "B" than your body secreting a complex series of hormones to balance mood and wellbeing. Although these are oversimplified descriptions, the function and the results are as real as they get.

As an analogy, we can think of ourselves as a spoiled rich kid. We have every advantage in life, and yet we refuse to use any of our innate or intrinsic gifts to provide for ourselves. Instead, we live off our parent's good graces until they cut us off. Once we cut ourselves off the "processed food inheritance," we become Steve Jobs - an unstoppable, creative force, efficient and powerful in manufacturing and meeting all your energy demands.

I think we all instinctively know that to be ultimately successful in weight-loss, we need to be on a journey to health. But we aren't going to settle for just health. No, we are reaching for the stars. After all, what good is health if we aren't happy? If we aren't happy, we *will* eventually seek out superficial and external stimuli in a futile attempt to find comfort. If that isn't the problem that society faces, I'll kiss your ass in public.

We have all willingly bought into a self-created illusion that despite overwhelming experiential evidence, we can somehow find a small measure of joy in a fleeting activity. Whether it be eating a fudge brownie that we know will leave us crashed and bloated an hour later or buying something on Amazon that gives us a rush of expectation only to be adorned to a nameless drawer after a few days. The same goes for playing video games or chasing after meaningless sex - we know these things won't bring us happiness. Yet, we allow a temporary illusion to exist where maybe, just maybe, we will get something different from the repeated experience. So, I guess what I'm saying is, addiction is a search for happiness with a really shitty sense of direction.

David Clark

Chapter 3
Who Am I?

"You cannot solve a problem from the same consciousness that created it. You must learn to see the world anew."
— *Albert Einstein*

"I am not nearly as smart as I think I am." That was the thought that saved my life. We all have had these thoughts or have said things like this before, but usually, it's more of a joke than an actual breakthrough. But it was real for me - I *meant* it, and it was a paradigm-busting moment of clarity. Strangely, my actual intelligence was irrelevant to the thought; the wisdom of the question lay in the fact that I finally stepped outside of the comfortable notion of my own competence. It was a break from the cover that certain areas of my life were giving me and being exposed to the hard reality of my blind spots moved the earth under my feet.

As a business owner, I was used to barking orders at people, dictating advertising strategies, and developing product lines that I knew people would buy. I was plugged into the heartbeat of my industry, and I was making a load of money because of it. But I wasn't *always* good at it, not always plugged in. I learned those things along with the slow evolution of my career as I went from part-time mattress salesman to owning my own chain of thirteen stores.

But as we humans grow, we tend to get complacent. We start to buy into our own press, and our own bullshit starts to smell less shitty until eventually, your whole outlook is based on the fleeting fragrance of past successes. When we experience a high level of accomplishment based on acquired wisdom in one area of focus, it can spill into our everyday life, creating blinding ignorance - at least it did for me.

The thought that I might not be as smart as I once imagined arrived because I was finally starting to see that when it came to my mattress business, I had things pretty well nailed down. But when it came to life - I was a monumental failure. Of course, eventually, it all came crashing down, as it does when you have a thousand plates spinning. I found myself on August 5, 2005, sitting on my bathroom floor at over three-hundred-twenty pounds, barely able to lift myself off the floor and into the shower. I was a raging alcoholic, and my medical symptoms read like a list of possible side effects for a prescription drug, "This lifestyle may cause drowsiness, vomiting, hallucinations, diabetes, restless leg syndrome, heart problems, and sudden death." The moment of clarity hit me like an asteroid collision changing the trajectory of my life forever. As it turns out, I wasn't a three-hundred-twenty-pound alcoholic by accident; after all, it was my thinking that got me there. It was my thinking that needed to change.

For years I operated under the illusion that some cosmic roll of the dice determined who I was.

David Clark

That my personality, ideas, faults, and tendencies were all a matter of how my DNA assembled itself. I didn't get the good-looking gene, didn't get the artist pedigree, but I did seem to catch onto things quickly, so I must be "the smart guy." I accepted that very thing as my identity early on in life. I'm sure it was based on little more than an errant compliment or two that I internalized. Maybe I did well on a couple of tests as a child, or maybe I felt some pride when I put together a puzzle a little faster than my brother. But somehow that one random idea caught a toehold in the myriad of feedback my young brain was receiving. Whatever it was, once I attached the idea of intelligence to the root of who I was, that gave me the leverage to ignore the times when I did dumb things. You know, like impaling myself on a sharp wooden post that I tried to leapfrog when I was ten.

Conversely, this identity anchor allowed me to burn into my memory the times I caught on to a new idea quickly or said something witty to the entertainment of my aunts and uncles. We all take our childhood traits and perceptions into our adult lives, and eventually, these narratives become powerful paradigms and foundational for how we navigate life. These bedrock notions eventually establish our limits, our comfort zones, and then without knowing it, they can become our prisons.

To ask someone "who are you?" will produce a broad spectrum of answers, and few of them are coherent, much less accurately descriptive. Some will cite their career choice as their identity. They may indicate that they are a police officer, or a teacher. Others might say "housewife" or "I'm just Julie." But who we are comes from a much deeper place than what we do, or even what our personalities quirks are. Who we are exists in the absence of all the people we know, all the things we have done, and even all the things we were taught. Who we are is something even more profound than our genetics. Who we are is more about energy or potential than it is our biology or background. Who we are is who we choose to be in the moment, or more accurately, how we choose to apply the malleable identity that existed in us before we were labeled with a name or an occupation. That's deep... hold on.

What I am saying is you are not your past. You are not your parents. It's closer to the truth to say who you are now is who you were *told to be* by the people around you, such *as* parents, teachers, and peers, as well as by yourself. At some point in your life who you *suspected* you might be, became who are you are now. Most of the time, this happened without us even being aware of the process. We just sort of slipped into our identity as if one day we tried on a comfortable set of shoes and later realized we never took them off. But I promise you that your identity is malleable. Those shoes can be kicked off. You can change everything about yourself. From how you think, to how you react, to how you look. So, if that's true, why do so many people fail when they try to change?

David Clark

In my experience, people don't fail because they aren't capable. They don't even fail because they aren't strong enough, they fail because they don't believe they can make it all the way to the end result. At some point along the way, they lose faith, the task starts to seem impossible, and they tap out with their best effort still inside. This happens for a few different but very specific reasons that we will go over in this chapter. But perhaps the biggest reason people don't succeed is they set themselves up for failure by not having a clear and *empowering* goal. When our goals aren't clear, we almost always fail to commit ourselves entirely to the effort.

Let's break down part of that equation - the failure part. Did you ever consider that there is no universal definition of failure? The only time we experience failure is when *we* define an experience as failure itself. To that point, we are consistently setting ourselves up to experience failure, by establishing arbitrary and sometimes insane rules.

Let's say I set a goal of losing weight; let's even make the goal more specific: I am going to lose one-hundred pounds. What do I do now? I further define my goal so that I have milestones to hit along the way - that makes sense. Small incremental change is the way, right? Okay, I would like to establish that my goal is to lose twelve pounds a month, three pounds a week. Sound familiar? It sounds tangible, right? I have a clear-cut goal, with specific benchmarks… Yet this is exactly how I set myself up to fail. I defined failure at the same time I defined my success. What happens if I diet hard, train my ass off, do everything right, and when I get on the scale, see that I didn't lose three pounds? What if instead I lost two pounds or God forbid only one pound? Has this happened to you? If so, did it feel like a failure? What actually happened in this scenario is you lost a pound. You are closer to the goal than you previously were, yet because you defined the rules so rigidly what should have been a success, now feels like a total disappointment.

I saw this with clients I trained at my gym day after day, month after month, year after year. I can still see them hanging their heads, a sick feeling in their gut, getting off the scale already defeated because they were certain that the effort they gave should have resulted in a five-pound loss of weight. They took no comfort in the fact they lost three pounds or even two; they were crushed.

The point is that we set ourselves up for failure by trying to control the very speed at which success will come. When we set our goals on things, we cannot control it, or we will eventually get punched in the face. What we *can* control is losing weight itself, getting leaner, and healthier. What we *cannot* control is what the exact number will be on the scale on any given day - that's insanity. Until we accept that failure exists only as a potential state of our own creation, we will repeat the cycle until one day we quit. The possibility of magically getting on the right program, with the perfect nutrition and experiencing the results in the precise predetermined rate of our guessing, is about as likely as me picking all six Powerball numbers next week.

Yet, there is a comfort to be found in the converse reality that we also get to choose what *success* is. In my life, I have learned to define success in one very specific way - *progress toward the goal*. Whatever my goal is, the focus is to continue to make progress in that direction. Sometimes there will be huge, quick strides in that direction, and at other times the progress is painfully and excruciatingly slow. But If I'm moving - I'm winning. Failure in my mind is defined *only* as quitting, walking away, or permanently giving up. I either win, or I learn. This is why, in my own weight-loss journey, I decided that the scale could no longer be the ultimate measure of my success. After all, hadn't I lost fifty pounds more than ten times, only to gain it all back? So, what good is the number anyway? Yes, I needed to make sure I was progressing toward my goal, but after having the scale rip my heart out so many times, I was willing to try something new.

Don't get the wrong impression, though I'm absolutely not about leaving our success to chance. I unequivocally think we must track our progress in any endeavor. We cannot be afraid to see where we are along the way and to make corrections as needed. I'm only saying we can't place a pass-fail on when and how the pounds will drop. In the end, I chose to take body measurements every week and only weigh myself once a month. If the measurements were going down - that was progress. I have discovered we aren't as emotionally attached to measurements as we are to weight, so it's a safer barometer by which we may track our progress.

Any movement on the tape measure was registered as good to me. A quarter of an inch lost sounds better to most people than losing a half-pound. This was a key factor in being able to stay on track and achieving my own long-term weight-loss. I believe that the reason I am here now at one-hundred-seventy pounds and not sitting at a McDonald's somewhere, is that my ultimate goal was not a number on the scale - it was health. It was total healing. Honestly (and perhaps ironically), I think ultimate health and healing is the only goal that will bring you the weight-loss number you seek. With healing your body as your goal, the number on the scale will come along for the ride, and you won't have to worry about maintaining it either - you'll just be there.

Later in this book, we will go into nutrition and what to eat to get results, but the truth is that all the diets I tried initially worked - right up until they didn't. I lost fifty pounds on South Beach, Atkins, Low-Fat, High-Fat, No Carbs; you name it. But those were just tricks, a set of rules, or a new dichotomy to make choices that would produce a temporary state. It was like I was "tricking" my body into losing weight by tricking my mind on what I was allowed to eat. But there was never a realistic chance that I would stay on those diets forever, so I was failing even as the pounds were coming off. To be successful in the long run, I had to change *me* before I changed my dinner plate.

So, with that in mind, before we even go over what you should be eating, let's get into how we can create an entirely "new you" first. You are going to need a new way of viewing yourself. You need to want to become the type of person that would never dream of eating the way you do now. You need to cast aside the old way of seeing things because if you don't, you will eventually go back to your old ways, even if you lose the weight.

I always thought of myself as the person who just couldn't lose weight. The unlucky and sad person with the painfully slow metabolism, predisposed to gaining weight, and sort of doomed to struggle with being heavy. I could see much evidence to support the theory. Even as an active youth playing baseball and riding my bike everywhere, I was fat. As a young adult, I wasn't afraid of taking off my shirt because I was modest, I was afraid of being called "ma'am." Insidiously, even when I had lost weight successfully in the past, there was always a pervasive feeling that I was spinning my wheels and that I would eventually gain it all back. Looking back now, I think I always hoped that if I could somehow, by hook or crook, get to my weight goal, the happiness of being skinny and attractive would be enough to convince me to stop overeating or somehow make me change my ways. But I was playing a game I would always lose.

There is nothing more powerful than who we think we are. If you view yourself as the type of person that always self-destructs, guess what happens when you get close to making something big happen? Yup, you blow it. If you think of yourself as an airhead, it's no shock to you when you try to unlock the front door to your house with your car key fob. But therein lies the illusion. We all do those things. We all self-destruct, we all walk into closed glass doors. Yet, not everyone considers doing something stupid as proof that they are of poor intelligence. The examples might seem like minor nuances, but these common everyday occurrences can become anchors for our identity and cause us to establish repeating preconditioned responses. This happens in both directions. Good or bad, positive reinforcement or negative.

If my deep internal concept of identity reflects one who is quite clever, should I lock my keys in my car? I simply laugh it off. I subconsciously ignore it as a fluke because it doesn't match my internal picture of self. I will do that EVERY time I lock the keys in the car for the rest of my life, even if I do it every day for a week. This is because, as humans, we continually ignore any information that conflicts with our identity while embracing anything that supports it.

Conversely, if I think of myself as an unintelligent person, and I deeply fear that people will learn of my shortcomings. What if I misunderstand the meaning of the company memo, and I hear my coworkers' laughter? It's immediately saved into my data bank as proof of my theory - cementing further

David Clark

and reinforcing my idea that I am dumb. It doesn't matter if five other people interpreted the memo as I did, my identity will predetermine the meaning.

Yet even the most obtuse of us cultivate brilliant ideas, and even the most eloquent speakers fumble over words at times. Einstein said, "We are all geniuses, but if you judge a fish by its ability to climb a tree, it will live its whole life, believing that it is stupid." I had a friend once tell me something very deep and insightful, and as I stood there taking in the brilliance of the idea, he quickly offered, "Oh, I must have heard that from someone else, I'm not that smart…" He was so uncomfortable standing in a place where someone viewed him as clever that he had to knock himself down to the level of his self-worth immediately. He was self-correcting a positive reinforcement *preemptively* because it didn't match his pre-programmed personality fingerprint.

We've all experienced these interactions, but now you *must* learn to become aware of these self-inflicted hatchet jobs if you are ever to move away from your old destructive self-communication. To fix your unwanted behaviors, you must adjust your internal self-portrait. You must become mindful of how you are interpreting reality around you if you hope to cultivate better internal awareness.

As I said previously, all concepts of identity start as a simple suggestion that made its way into our subconscious. Maybe your parents said you were the musical one, or maybe you were told you are "unusually determined" or curious. Or maybe you were even told that you would never amount to anything. Whatever suggestion you received, good or bad that landed on your psyche, stayed in your thoughts until it eventually wormed its way into your subconscious mind. At some point, you started giving that little angel or demon some rental space. For a while, you fought back on it, you doubted it, and you turned it over endlessly until one day you started to explore the substance of it. Did it make sense? Does it fit into the pictures stored in your mind? At some unknown point you started to believe it. You no longer suspected it might be true, it *became* true - you made it true. You kicked that teetering loose brick back into the wall so hard it lodged itself firmly in your foundation and became real. With a seamless transition, your mind continued its job as the ultimate computer, constantly saving and deleting data to support its new operating parameters.

Many people have made the analogy that our minds are computers, and this is profoundly true as it relates to identity. Like computers, our minds are constantly saving and deleting information. If on your laptop computer you kept every photo, program, and stored document you ever viewed, the computer would become useless. Instead, we have to choose what information is important enough to save, so our computers don't become too full to operate. This is exactly how our brain chooses which memories and thoughts to encode deeply. When presented with information, your mind-computer goes through a simple check: Does this support our self-identity

David Clark

concept? If the answer is yes - it saves it. If the answer is no - it deletes it. It's that simple. After a long enough period of time, and a multitude of experiences, you have saved enough information that your identity has grown very strong. It has now become a core belief with voluminous data to support it. It no longer matters if you experienced an equal or greater number of life experiences that would have stood in direct contrast to your identity; those are gone and never recorded. What you are left with is a one-sided argument, constructed on emotional and anecdotal bullshit.

From this powerful new paradigm, you navigate your life. All your decisions, choices, hobbies, and relationships are all run through the cipher. Should something significant occur, say, getting fired, the end of a relationship, or anything that causes you to question your idea of who you are… The internal argument eventually fails to see the light of day as its standing in the shadow of a myriad of tainted evidence.

Another way that our minds are like computers is that they cannot engage in conflicting operations. If you program your computer to reduce your electricity consumption by giving it access to all your appliances and lights and then install a different program that will keep all the lights on for twenty-four hours a day, seven days a week, something will break. The internal conflict will eventually create a fatal system error. Similarly, you cannot simply choose to live a peaceful or happy life when your actions, beliefs, and behaviors are in conflict.

Pre-programmed into the human mind is the need for how we act to match who we think we are. Case in point, if a man considers himself to be a moral man, a Christian man, if his very identity is tied into a sense of him being a good father and servant of God… I am not talking about someone trying to *convince* himself or others of who he is, but the person that truly believes this is who they are. This person has lived a life of service, fidelity, and pious action. If this person in a moment of weakness, perhaps while inebriated, or after experiencing an emotional breakdown, has a marital affair, he will be in total conflict with himself. He will pace the floor, become stressed, and he may find himself unable to sleep or focus at work. He will literally become tormented by his own mind as he drives himself nuts with constant guilt. He may end up confessing his sins to his wife, his pastor, or he may even live in conflict for the rest of his life, destroying his peace of mind until relief finally comes on his death bed as he releases the burden he has been carrying.

Conversely, if a different man who has no such idea of morality attached to himself engages in the same behavior, there will be no conflict if he views himself as a hustler, someone that lives by his own rules, a playboy, a bad boy, someone not tied to society's values. If this man has random sex with a married woman, there is no personal crisis at all. This is very real, and it happens all the time. Astonishingly,

David Clark

people like this, seemingly good people, leave their lovers' beds every day and go immediately home for dinner with their spouse and kids without missing a beat. They kiss the kids and talk about how their day went with their significant other with no turmoil. No nagging voices, no crisis. Why? Because the behavior doesn't create a conflict with the internal concept of self... The man knows deep inside he cannot be trusted; he knows the rules of fidelity don't apply to him. The mind creates no conflict because there isn't one. So, either the actions have to change, or the identity has to change for homeostasis or internal calmness to exist.

The human need to be devoid of internal conflict also applies to your own particular struggle with food. If you think of yourself as the type of person that cannot lose weight, or someone that will always struggle with gaining weight, or someone who just loves eating cupcakes, you will always be in conflict when you try to change any behavior that lives inside that identity. When the diet gets hard, when the cupcakes look good enough, you will go back. You will say, "Who am I kidding? This isn't me; I'll never be able to do this." Just like that, you are back at rock bottom. Who we believe ourselves to be is the gateway to all the things we do, good or bad, small or large.

We all get caught in cycles of bad behavior that we can't break. Many times, we even make feeble attempts to eliminate the conflict by bending our self-image to fit the new behavior. But this falls short of a true identity change. This is only to grant permission to ourselves to continue to indulge in old habits in hopes that we can sleep better at night. The alcoholic might say, "I am going to become a writer because writers are alcoholics, and I can drink every day while I write." Or we can say, "I am going to be a swimmer so I can eat like Michael Phelps." But this is only a bridge loan. You haven't really solved the problem; you've only granted a temporary illusion that the mind chooses to buy into. Eventually, it all comes crumbling down and leaves us broken and unable to have any peace of mind. Let's its face it, you didn't really want to train like Phelps; you were just hungry. You didn't really want to torture yourself in front of a computer for two years trying to write *A Farewell to Arms* either, you just wanted to get drunk on a Tuesday.

When I tried unsuccessfully to lose weight in the past, I always collided head-on with "Big Dave," that lovable but tragically sad clown I viewed myself as. He loved to eat, to cook, and to live life! What bullshit. I used to talk about how much I loved the McRib at the same time I spoke of gourmet dinners, one-hundred-dollar Kobe steaks, and two-thousand-dollar bottles of wine. Sometimes I did this while eating Taco Bell... Talk about trying to bend the picture of who you are. After almost twenty years of the back and forth self-loathing battle raging inside me, eventually, I had to let go. I permanently deleted the old picture of myself like a scorned lover catches fire to the last remaining photo of their ex. It was scary, but I knew I had to do it.

Let me ask you a question… what do you think your chances are of making a long-term change if the essence of how you think remains unchanged? If you answered zero, you are right. You must become willing to let go of the old you. You must become willing to be broken and vulnerable to be able to rebuild. I know that might sound scary, especially if you bought this book with the comfortable idea that you like who you are. But I challenge you to go deeper. Try to touch briefly, right now, that part of you that knows deep down inside there is something toxic in how you eat. Something you fear that might be hidden in you. Just reach out for a second and see if it's there… if you can't see it or aren't willing to - you should probably take a little break from reading and come back when you can see it. But if you find it and if you stick around, I'll show you how to unpack all that fear in the **Radical Rehab**, and I'll help you slay those demons in the process. Oh, and you won't lose who you are in this program. Actually, you'll find just how amazing you are underneath all that pain and fear you are carrying.

Okay, all this sounds great, but how the hell do you do it? How do you change who you are? I am going to make it as straightforward as I know how - you become the person you want to be. Now - for no good reason. You don't go on a journey. You don't go on a search to find the best version of you. You choose who you want to be now. You throw yourself into that life and burn the fucking bridge behind you - leave no opportunity for retreat. You can do that; I promise you can.

When I was sitting at the rock bottom of my life, I was broke because I had pissed away millions of dollars. I had high blood pressure, a heart condition, and a drug and alcohol addiction as big as Texas. I was broken down as a man. I had no confidence; I couldn't follow through on a single promise, not one. I couldn't return a phone call, I couldn't walk to the mailbox, I couldn't do a single thing. But I stand before you today as an entirely different human.

My athletic accomplishments include running some of the toughest ultramarathons on the planet. I have run the Boston Marathon four times in one day, I have run for forty-eight hours straight on a treadmill, and I have become the athlete that I always dreamt of being, which is the kind of athlete I always respected from my old bar stool. That means that all those tears I shed in embarrassment when I walked down the aisles of planes seeing people look away hoping to God, I didn't sit next to them. All those times I cried in the mirror or hid in shame from my own indulgent behaviors. All the times I felt I was trapped in a bloated and failing shell of a body was all based on bullshit. It was a lie. I sold myself huge lies - that I was born fat and that I was born to fail. That no matter what I did, I could never escape the truth of who I was – it was all bullshit. Hopefully, I am

David Clark

bringing home the point that I was wrong about everything, including who I was, and so are you.

If you accept the reality that who you think you are is wrong, then you will no longer feel trapped, or destined to fail. You were not born to be where you are now. You were not born to be overweight, depressed, or addicted to anything. Fourteen years ago, I grabbed hold of a thought, and I never let it go. The thought was, "Maybe I wasn't supposed to be a three-hundred-twenty-pound alcoholic." What if I was supposed to be an athlete, and I just messed it up? Hell, it made sense to think that I screwed up who I was supposed to be. Why not?

I screwed everything else up. Here is the most important part of it all… from that moment on, I chose to believe something new. For me, the new image was being a runner, a marathon runner to be more specific. Just like a child starting from scratch, I had to embark on a brand new journey. I had to believe in something crazy. So, I did, from one thought to the next. Each thought was the gateway to the next thought. I had to let go of the past entirely and learn to believe in the future, even in the face of doubt. Having the willingness to do that, just might have saved my life - it certainly changed it.

Obviously, at three-hundred-twenty pounds, the new "marathon version of me" didn't have a lot of clout in the internal courtroom of my consciousness. I was quite sure I was full of shit. Being a smart-ass New Yorker, I kind of felt like a District Attorney sitting at the other table each time I threatened to introduce evidence that the old me no longer had tenure. "I object!" My subconscious would say that every time I passed up Burger King for a Subway Veggie Delight. "This man loves Beanie Weenees, and he isn't a vegetarian!" My mind would rage against me when I woke up early to go to the gym. "This isn't who we are!" But I put my head down and did the work. I created a new life that was more powerful than the objections and more enticing than the idea of staying fat and broken.

If all this seems confusing or a bit much, it's okay. I am going to spell it out for you in the ten steps that you will be doing later. But I need you to be willing to take the same plunge that I did. The same level of commitment is required for everyone that wants to make the change. Later in the **Radical Rehab,** you will need to place a completely new identity as the dichotomy for everything you do moving forward. Every choice you make has to be run through the precept of the "new you." What you choose to eat, what you choose to wear, what movies you watch, and even how you sit on the couch, everything has to be sent through the wash cycle. "How does this new person relax?" "What does someone who gives a fuck about health purchase at the grocery store?" Now, this might sound quite insane, and make no mistake, it is. But I am laying the groundwork in this chapter for the real substantive work that is coming… you didn't think this was just another recipe book, did you?

David Clark

As a weight-loss professional, I tend to get the same questions all the time: What do I need to do to change? Should I switch to Keto? Intermittent fasting? Vegan? Starvation? But I am going challenge you to ask a different question, a better question. Let's worry less about what behavior you should change and focus on asking: Who do you want to be? What is the life you want to live?

I am not trying to make you become a runner, let's get that out of the way now in case you were shifting uncomfortably in your chair for the last thirty minutes. I could not care less about who you choose to become or whether you ever run a mile in your life. Over the years, I have helped hundreds of people lose weight and change themselves. Some of them chose to be runners, some triathletes, some community health advocates, cross-fitters, bowlers, or day-hikers. It doesn't matter what you choose to become as long as you choose something emotionally attractive to *you,* and that has total body health in its gravitational pull.

In *my* new identity, I was committed to becoming an athlete. The type of athlete that wouldn't dream of eating double Quarter Pounders for breakfast or show up drunk for brunch. I romanticized it. I fell in love with the idea of a new life. I needed to make sure I wanted that new life bad enough to get leverage on myself to follow through, to be willing to walk away from my old life completely. I had to want to be a new guy so bad that I was willing to do or believe anything to get there. The new picture wasn't just a leaner, fit body. It was health, happiness, and a feeling of accomplishment that I was chasing too. That is exactly what it takes to change. You have to want the "new" more than you are afraid of the pain of changing. You have to own the want itself and cultivate the desire. You have to want a new life, and you have to be willing to prove you want it when it comes time to do the work. You can't break food addiction by passively wanting to "eat better." So, take this to heart now, and adjust your goals accordingly if you aren't chomping at the bit to live a whole new life by now.

Hopefully, you are already there, and you want this change badly. But, if not, you can learn to want it too. One of the keys to learning, to really want something is to make sure you have completely let go of the past way of doing things. I hear people all the time say, "Well, it could always be worse." I hate this statement because although it's designed to be an exercise in gratitude, it ignores the obvious fact that things could be a hell of a lot better. If you look around, you might notice that being overweight kind of sucks. It sucks to be embarrassed at how you look, and to be a slave to fried and sugary foods. It sucks always to be worried about how much fat is showing, narrow seats, beach parties, and anything else that shouldn't be a big deal. Before the "politically correct" police start flogging me, I'm not saying that the worth of a person lays solely in their physical appearance, I am stating the simple truth that being overweight is a fixable condition that almost everyone would choose to fix if they thought it was possible. Just like you feel better when you put on a nice looking sweater or hat, can you imagine how much better it feels when your body feels and looks better, and is providing you a higher level of energy? Fucking amazing. That's how it feels.

When you dare to touch the pain of your current life deeply, two things happen: You become grounded to the reality of where you are, and you clearly identify a specific area that you want to improve. The Buddha said one of the keys to ending suffering in our lives is to hold our pain like a child. To feel it and (this is key) to let it go. Hiding from the pain of being overweight gives it power it doesn't deserve. To confront obesity head-on provides us with the commitment to move away from it. When the pain of staying where we are becomes greater than the pain of moving forward - we change. So, take some time right now to really feel the burden your current life is inflicting on you. Feel the embarrassment, the feeling of failure, the hopelessness. I want to make sure you know what is at stake here.

One of the biggest myths I see perpetuated is the notion that fit and active people are just naturally motivated to train. But in my experience, the most motivated people in the world are the ones that constantly work on being motivated. Let me say that again - the driven person is not necessarily born with an inherent drive. Motivation is not a genetic trait - it's the result of hard work. Constantly stoking the fire, feeding the flame, and touching the goal in every moment. When a professional fighter is cutting weight before a fight, they have the best filter in the world to choose what to eat: Will this help me make weight and win this fight, or will it make it more likely that I lose?

To stay motivated throughout this rehab, you should develop the habit of asking yourself if what you are doing supports building a new life? We ask ourselves this question because it brings us to simple choices: Yes or no? This or that? Will this make me stay the way I am or help me become the person I want to be? It's got to be one or the other. This keeps the vision sharp and eliminates all that gray area where we engage in things we haven't clearly defined as good or bad. As you can probably see, these questions are of particular importance to the act of eating. It puts us squarely in the moment and mindful of all our food choices.

This kind of focus keeps us on the cutting edge of the reasons we are doing all of this - to create a new life. We need to continue establishing this connection over and over again (especially early on) to keep the fire burning. If we lose touch, we can slip into old habits without even being aware of it. Nothing is worse than realizing you threw away your new life halfway through a pizza. If you can engage in this mindful practice for long enough, it will become so routine that you won't even notice it. It will be like driving to work in the morning or drinking a cup of coffee - just something you do by habit.

David Clark

As we have visited earlier in the book, one of the biggest reasons we overeat is because we have lost the connection with how food affects us. We eat when we're bored. We eat poorly ten minutes after we promise ourselves that we aren't going to eat junk anymore. Have you ever felt yourself getting up from the chair and going into the kitchen, grabbing a bowl of cereal, and eating it almost as if you weren't controlling your body? Like you were just along for the ride, watching as the action unfolds? Hoping you will eat the junk food and also hoping you will talk yourself out of it at the same time? This happens for a very simple but complicated reason. Your body is a survival machine, and although it's capable of accomplishing monumentally difficult acts, it will choose the path of least resistance whenever left to its own devices. This is why we have been given command over our impulses with our advanced consciousness. No other animal can question itself or choose to change what it believes.

If we as humans weren't able to do the things that we didn't want to do, we would die. We wouldn't work, gather food, socialize, or keep our bodies strong. Plus, we would all kill our children within the first five years of their lives, thereby eliminating the human race. The point is we now know that once our bodies become aware that fried chicken and bread exist, it will generally prefer to eat that as opposed to converting its own fat to energy. If it has to shortcut your consciousness to get it, well, it may do just that. The good news is the human body has a shitty memory. Once it forgets about crappy processed food, it won't try to trick you into eating it again. But to break the cycle, you have to commit to rewiring your brain to be aware of everything you are putting in your mouth.

What I need you to internalize before we move on is that this new picture of who you are needs to be connected to all that you are doing. Every thought, every action, and all your motivations. If you do this right, it should be fun. Relate your journey to characters that inspire you in movies, picture yourself doing the things they are doing, the types of things you've dreamt off. Allow yourself to take on role models and inspirational mentors. We all need this. The greatest athletes and leaders all engage and indulge themselves in allowing their dreams to seep into their daily actions and motivations. It's ok to visualize winning the New York City Marathon even on your first slow and painful runs. It's ok to picture being on top of Everest or swimming the English Channel.

One day, it'll become real. Maybe not exactly as you picture it, but a version of it will be real. All the things that seemed so outlandish for me years ago can now be found on my Instagram feed. As for the people that would make you feel childish about dreaming of becoming an athlete as an overweight person later in life, they are the ones that aren't getting the results you want. Listen only to the people that are standing where you want to be. All, and I mean *ALL* the great people I have had the privilege of

David Clark

meeting are the ones that understand there is no wisdom in the flock. You must be willing to do the things nobody else is doing if you want the results no one gets.

Much of the focus of the **Radical Rehab** you will be doing is designed to help you rewire your thinking. One of the things we will be working on is becoming mindful while you eat. Have you heard the expression that your body is a temple? Well, I'm going to take it one step further - I want you to make eating a religious experience. Commune with it. Worship your food, cherish your food, put all your love into your food. Make the experience of eating as sensory and mindful as possible. Be aware of the weight of the fork in your hand. Feel the texture of the veggies as your teeth slowly chew, and your tongue tastes. Try to experience every individual thing on your plate. Take note of your feet touching the floor, the sensation of your food as it makes its way into your stomach.

This might sound crazy, but you will actually change not just the way your brain interacts with the eating process, but you will also activate your consciousness to the process of nourishment. This mind-body connection has a profound and measurable effect on all physiological and physical activities. Any trainer will tell you that the athlete who gets to the gym and runs through the motions of a workout will have a profoundly different effect than the athlete that is aware of the purpose of every rep as they feel the muscle move and contract. Show your body how important eating is for you, and it will return the favor by craving healthy, healing choices. After all, that is the goal, right? To stop craving the junk that you are currently living off of.

Now so that you know, you will fail horribly at this mindful stuff. That's kind of the point, in a way. At first, you will eat on autopilot and then remember to be mindful after the fact. Don't get mad. Next time be ready. Next time you'll likely forget what you are doing after a few seconds of mindful eating, but then you'll remember and try to get reconnected. But the process of being aware that you aren't totally present in eating is itself part of being mindful. The first stages of your practice will just be *being aware you aren't being aware.* You will eventually fall in deeper, and it will happen without thinking about it.

Just like the runner that one day realizes they can hardly go a day without running despite hating it for a year - you won't even think of mindful eating as anything other than eating. While you are practicing being present for the act of eating, try being present in the act of planning *what* to eat too. Make healthy, vibrant food a priority in your life. Embrace the act of preparing your foods. That doesn't mean that you have to become a full-time chef, but thinking like one is a move in the right direction.

Plan your meals, even if you are planning on eating on the run. Picture living, bright, healthy, healing foods when you are hungry. Although we will get more into the nuts and bolts of food choices in my ten-step rehab plan, I want you to start changing your thinking now - before we even dig in.

As you already know, all the planning, promises, and intentions to eat healthy, don't mean shit if they never make it to becoming habit. Have you ever made a promise to yourself and then prayed to God that you would keep it? As if you didn't have everything you need to keep the promise yourself? But that shows where we are sometimes. It's as if we think a healthy and fit body will come by chance or divine intervention. Or maybe we hope we will figure out how to make the kind of commitment that is so deep that it can keep itself. Like we could somehow commit hard enough that our minds will magically change. Sorry, that's not a commitment, that's wishful thinking.

But I can share how you will know if you have made a *real* commitment to change - It will be followed immediately by an action. The bigger the action, the bigger your commitment is. There is absolutely no such thing as a commitment that isn't followed by an action. If you make an internal choice to change something, you will HAVE to do something; you won't be able to sleep if you don't. Because in the presence of commitment, the passive comfort of a soft promise is dead. A shallow resolution might give you a temporary respite from the struggle, but you will never feel continuing peace from simple assertions. True freedom comes in knowing that you are actually bringing about the change. So, if you find yourself going through the motions of the action plan later in this book, but not doing the work, STOP immediately and go back. Do not be one of the people that lets this program sit unused on your nightstand like a winning lottery ticket never cashed in.

Finally, I caution you to resist the impulse to attempt to make this program easy. There is no easy path to change. There is no easy way to lose weight. Well, that's not entirely true. Ironically the only easy way to lose weight is to stop trying to make it easy. When we back into a challenge, we will never rise to the occasion. I've seen so many people (myself included) try to jump into weight-loss with the goal of making it as painless as possible. We search for the right plan, diet, or trick that seems the least intrusive, all with the hopes that this new direction will somehow produce results - bullshit.

Results never come from easy action. Nothing great or difficult is ever done in the comfort zone. Can you imagine an MMA fighter stepping in the cage with a game-plan designed to make the confrontation as painless as possible? To fight, you have to impose your will on the opponent. You have to be the one dictating the pace and action. And so, it is the same with this journey to becoming the ultimate you. For this fight, you must be the one calling the shots, pushing hard into the challenge, and owning the pain of the struggle. I learned to relish my hunger when I was losing weight. If I went to bed at night feeling I wanted to eat more, it was a victory. When I chose to eat an apple instead of a candy bar, I felt empowered, encouraged. When you embrace the fact that this is a fight, you might just smile as the punches come.

That means that every time you confront the remnants of the old you, the one that wants to give in, don't lay back and wonder how long this fight will last. Stand up and say, "I am in control of what I eat!" I have literally shouted that from the top of my lungs into the mirror when my mind was cluttered up. Do you want to feel motivated? Try looking right into the mirror and telling the demons to go fuck themselves.

Years ago, I was on a twenty-mile training run with some people from a local running group. Apparently, there was some chat about my weight-loss story. At the end of the run, one of the runners who only knew me as "the guy that runs one-hundred-mile races" said, "Dude, I heard you used to weigh three-hundred-twenty pounds… is that right?"

"Yup," I said back.

"You know that's considered impossible by many people, right? How the hell did you get from there to here?"

Without thinking, I kind of laughed and said, "If I would have known how hard it was going to be - I'd have done it sooner." That was it. It kind of fell out of my mouth, but it was the single most relevant thing I ever said about how weight-loss is done. "Rise to the challenge, do the hard things, believe in yourself." If you do that, your body will show you all the strength you never knew it had. By taking this offensive approach to your own journey, not only will you activate your personal strength and power, but you will actually become stronger in the process. Yes, by being aggressive in this process, you will be more prepared to live life moving forward once you hit your weight-loss goal. This prophecy is self-fulfilling. You will wake up one morning and realize that you hit your weight goal months or even years ago, and it didn't even register as a special day - it was a simple "today."

David Clark

Chapter 4
Prescription Meditation

*"I'm not a New Age person, but I do believe in
meditation, and for that reason I've always liked the
Buddhist religion."*
— Clint Eastwood

If you're like me, you think meditation is some
hippie bullshit, self-indulgent pompous posturing that
only the shallowest humans would pretend to be
interested in. Previously, when I heard the word
"meditation," I would see a robe-clad bearded dirtbag
sitting on a big cushion with circular purple glasses
saying "ooooommmm" perhaps dreaming of Ultimate
Frisbee. But then I heard about the Vedas and The
Shaolin Monks. I read *The Bhagavad Gita* and
encountered glorious stories of ancient warriors
sitting in meditation sometimes for days, weeks, and
months at a time as they prepared for battle or tried to
transcend the limits of their earthly bodies. I became
absolutely enamored with the relationship between
attempting impossible feats of strength and
endurance-based activities solely based on mental or
spiritual acuity.

There is an undeniable mystic or curiosity
surrounding meditation. Underneath my initial
cynicism, there *was* a genuine curiosity about the
practice and what it might be able to deliver. Maybe it
hits on the deep-seated desire we all have in order to

unlock the hidden power of the human mind. We are told from a young age that we only use ten percent of our brains. We have been influenced by movies like "The Matrix" or "Limitless" that suggest regular humans can become superhuman if they can only find a mechanism to strip away the layers that society has placed over their perceptions. We all feel like we would benefit from a break from the never-ending inner voices, doubts, and fears that plague us as we move about throughout our days.

But if you are like most people, you probably have several failed attempts at meditation. Have you felt something akin to intense pressure or anxiety from simply trying to sit and be alone in silence? Me, too. Which, oddly, is proof that we need to meditate, not proof that we can't. The Dalai Lama once famously said, "Everyone should meditate for at least ten minutes every day unless you are too busy in which case you should do twenty minutes."

Writing this today, I can say that meditation *has* had a profound effect on my personal transformation. Not just in becoming an accomplished athlete, but to ending my battles with food addiction and to restoring my mind to a state of almost perpetual peace. From my anxiety-filled, overthinking childhood to my manic, unrelenting, unyielding, and controlling adult addiction tendencies, a calm and relaxed man has emerged from the meditation cushion. I still get stressed, I still experience fear, of course, but my practice has allowed me to draw on an internal source of instant

David Clark

peace. It's allowed me to let go of destructive thoughts, instantly release panic, and remain calm while everyone else around me is losing their shit.

But before I tell you why meditation is a part of the **Radical Rehab**, let's talk about what it is. In its most remedial form, it's a break. A reset. A way to interrupt the non-stop bombardment of inner voices and thoughts. It's a chance for your central processing unit to reboot and install updates. Do you remember when we talked about our minds being like computers? If you can indulge me, think of the modern human as a computer that has never closed the open windows of its mind. It has thousands of webpages and programs running at all times. Sorry, but that's you, and it used to be me, too.

Today's chaotic lifestyles place tremendous draw on the processing capability of our brains. Yes, we are capable of processing an undeniably large amount of data, but not without cost. Irritability, frustration, and loss of focus make it almost impossible to access any of the software available to us as humans to be calm, creative, and efficient in our daily lives. Instead we stumble about our days trying to sort through the sea of open programs in our minds, unable to execute any one thing at a high level. The result is that nothing gets done well enough to move on. Instead we open window after window in the form of new work projects, unresolved conflicts, and impending crisis management, all adding to the already diminished capacity of our mental energy stores. So… in its most functional form, think of meditation as a reboot. It's closing all the open programs and resetting your mind so that it can focus on what tasks need to be done.

At first, meditation doesn't need to be anything more than just sitting and breathing. It's giving all of your resources over to a simple task - being present. Meditation is being still in a comfortable place. Preferably a quiet place, trying only to be aware of your body as you breathe in and out with intention. Although it's a simple effort, it is nonetheless serious business, and you will do well to treat it as such. In that regard, make sure you prepare a specific place to meditate. It can be in a guest room, in the den, the living room, or wherever you think will provide you the best uninterrupted and sensory devoid environment. I suggest meditating at the same time each day, either first thing in the morning or at the end of the day. Do not meditate while lying down. Sit upright, with a straight back and relaxed hands and feet. I will go over the physical aspects and process for meditation in the rehab plan, but for now, start to think of this as something that deserves your intention.

Meditation is a tool we are going to use, but it doesn't have to have an agenda. It doesn't have to even have a purpose yet. You cannot "succeed" or "fail" at it. For now, the act of sitting and breathing only needs to be something that you are willing to do and something that you are trying to be totally aware of while doing it. If you choose to continue in the

David Clark

practice of meditation long-term, you will find the practice itself changes and flourishes as you evolve.

Think of these early days of meditation as sitting on the bench while learning to play the piano. At first, you will be painfully pressing one key at a time as your mind struggles to make internal associations of which key provides what sound. It will be frustrating at times; you will feel untalented, and the process itself might even seem futile. But one day, the keys will become notes instead of random sounds. You will start to hear the noises as parts of something bigger. You will learn to blend separate notes into rich and textured chords. Eventually, your mind will cease even to be aware of your hands or the piano itself, and one day you will be walking in a beautiful song that is springing forth underneath your fingertips, courtesy of the deliberate effort of those early lessons.

I'm sure you have guessed by now that mediation is going to be a part of your rehab. Ironically, if that stresses you out, consider it proof that you would benefit greatly from learning the practice. But why? Why should you just wholesale buy into the idea that meditation will change how you eat? Let's dig in…

As a trainer and coach who has worked with hundreds of overeaters - and from my own experience as a three-hundred-pound puppy myself - I can say it's the *mindless* eating that is the most devastating. I remember many times being ten days or more into a diet or weight-loss program that was working well, only to self-destruct myself for no reason. One minute I was looking in the mirror, proud of the noticeable change in my profile, the next I was eating a triple-decker PB&J wondering what happened. It was like a separate entity took control of my body, walked into the kitchen, grabbed three slices of bread, and started to assemble the medicine. I could feel a certain amount of panic rising inside. It was an insane mixture of both wanting to talk myself out of eating the delicious food, while at the same time telling myself to shut the fuck up before I ruined it for myself.

Perhaps the most relevant thing meditation can do for us overeaters is to provide a relationship between our actions and exactly what we want. What we *truly* want. As previously stated, on a root level, all of our behaviors, desires, and actions stem from a desire to be happy. The problem is we live in a world where we have loose and disconnected notions of what *happy* is. Certainly, being healthy, fit, and lean will make us feel good. But so will that tub of ice cream. The brain gets confused between the two conflicting paths, and in the presence of conflict, it's the simple, quick fix that usually wins. This is why it is so important to cultivate a healthy and compelling relationship with a long-term desire. Our minds are quite proficient at delivering an outcome when we direct our intention to a specific goal, but that same brain sputters and stalls when given vague and unconnected goals.

David Clark

The runner who makes their goal "I want to be fast" might get some result from training. But the runner who says, in six months from now on May 10th, I want to run a "10k" averaging a five-minute, fifty-seven-second pace, will have a vastly different experience. The brain snaps to attention at the laser-sharp goal. It starts to work backward and calculate the volume of running required. It allocates time, schedules, and training markers needed to run such a race. The runner with "fast" as the goal may also change their training in response, but it will be loose and fragmented. It will be hard to get motivated for such a vague goal, and the runner will likely fail to achieve the experience they desire.

It's obvious that most of us move from task to task throughout the day without ever being truly aware of what we are doing. We wake up, we immediately put on a pot of coffee, start the shower, get dressed, jump in the car, and drive to work as if it were one event. We blend every aspect of our daily life into one twenty-four-hour block. These twenty-four-hour blocks are used to build a three-sixty-five-day brick that fits into the wall of our lives. But each year, each day, each hour or minute is unto itself a lifetime. Remember, our minds are very good when given a specific task to accomplish, which makes it a tragedy that so few of us ever give our undivided attention to any one thing.

Imagine if tomorrow you simply broke down your day into individual experiences. If you were present completely while you made coffee. If you took a deep breath before you got dressed. If you transformed your drive to work into an experience worth enjoying, can you imagine how much more effective you'd be on that day? Can you already picture yourself arriving at work more energized, more prepared to have a creative and energized day? I would submit that the stress of the daily grind would not have a hold over you on that day. Your own energy would override the drab and lifeless actions of others.

How different would your health be if you were present in all your behaviors, including how you eat? Meditation is going to help you clear out all the ambiguity in your relationship with food, eating, and health. It is going to help clear the way for you to be mindful and aware of how all your actions affect your health as a goal. It will help you to establish a direct line of communication with your higher self. The same self that knows eating a cupcake is ten seconds of joy and a week of regret. Notice I said meditation will *help* you. I did not say it would deliver these promises without effort. Consider meditation to be a performance-enhancing drug - you still have to turn the pedals if you want to win the "Tour de France."

You can see that I want you to take the mediation part of my program very soberly. That is because I want you to succeed at this. I want you to learn to put an end to this terrible spiral that destructive foods have put you on. You are not alone on this journey - I am personally invested in your success. Because of that, I ask for no less than your

David Clark

one-hundred percent commitment to meditate. I don't give a shit if you don't want to. I am sure you don't want to continue on this path of eating yourself to death, either.

So, give yourself to this completely. Think of this as a spiritual pilgrimage. A quest of the new warrior that will emerge thirty days from now. Take pride in the ritual of meditation, layer it into a bigger picture of how it can help you. Be humble, do the things you previously would have scoffed at. But remember, this takes time. We are learning to play the piano. You cannot *will* yourself to be Mozart in one day, you can only will yourself to endure the practice sessions until the concerto comes.

Chapter 5
Food Is Our Medicine

"You have just dined, and however scrupulously the slaughterhouse is concealed in the graceful distance of miles, there is complicity."
— *Ralph Waldo Emerson*

More good news: You are going to be plant-based for the next thirty days. Glad to see you made it back to your chair, I hope the fall didn't hurt you. If you don't know what plant-based is, don't worry, I'll explain. But first, let me tell you something that's going to be hard to hear - humans aren't natural meat-eaters. I know, I know. I'm not saying you *can't* eat meat - obviously, you can. I'm only saying it's really hard on our human bodies to process meat, at least to the extent and quantity that the American diet delivers it. But we are going to keep this small. Thirty days small, to be exact. So I am not going to be asking you to "go vegan for the animals." I am only asking, scratch that, demanding, okay, okay... *asking* that you commit to putting only whole plant-based foods into your body during this healing period. I'll explain why, but for now, think of it as a cleanse.

It seems like the words "Whole-Food Plant-Based" (WFPB) are bounced around all over Facebook, Netflix, and practically every discussion about nutrition these days. But many people are still very unsure what makes up a whole-food, plant-based diet. In simple terms, a WFPB diet excludes any meat, poultry, fish, dairy, or eggs while it emphasizes a large variety of whole foods. The term "whole" in WFPB describes foods that are minimally processed. This includes eating as many whole grains, fruits, vegetables, and legumes as you desire. It also includes nuts, seeds, avocados, natural sweeteners, and certain soy or wheat products that don't contain added fat such as tofu, tempeh, and seitan.

Heavily processed foods, however, are not included in a WFPB diet. This means avoiding refined grain products such as white rice, white flour, and foods containing added sugars or artificial sweeteners. That's it, at least for the purposes of your **Radical Rehab**. Many people debate endlessly on the nuances of the diet and add various rules such as no oil, no sweeteners, etc. Trust me, people can always complicate things. It's what humans are best at. I'll be going much deeper into food choices during the program, but if you stick to the basics I line up for you, you will not just lose the pounds, you will heal your broken body, and that is why we are here.

Don't worry, you won't need a calculator or a food scale. You don't have to excessively count calories or weigh your food (although there is a five-day calorie-restrictive phase). Don't believe the people that tell you convenience is your enemy. You can do a WFPB plan from anywhere in the world, even while traveling, working eighty hours a week, or whatever your lifestyle is.

You certainly won't be learning to grow beets or lettuce in the backyard in this program. You are allowed frozen fruits and vegetables if it is needed (just make sure to find no-preservatives or additives versions). I do, however, suggest fresh produce and veggies as much as humanly possible. Oh, and blandness is not a prerequisite either. You're encouraged to experiment with as many spices as you'd like.

Finally, contrary to popular belief, a WFPB diet won't break your budget. Many of your trusted staples (think beans and potatoes) are among the most affordable foods in the grocery store. This diet doesn't require specialty items hidden in the health food section. It requires no sprouted mung beans, tofu, or shopping carts full of cashews (although those things are all awesome).

As for the other benefits of not eating animal products, I wrote an entire chapter on my own personal Buddhist, Libertarian reasons for going plant-based in my book *Broken Open,* so I won't hit you with all of that. Still, I do want to put some context into why I am asking you do go plant-based for *this* program. I can assure you it has more to do with your health than it does your politics.

Let's get started by addressing a few of the myths surrounding vegans and plant-based diets in general. What is a "vegan" anyway? In "The Simpsons, " I think it was the bartender Moe that said a "level five" vegan is someone who won't eat anything that casts a shadow... Hmm, seems extreme, and sometimes I think that might be where it's heading, and although funny, it does show where mainstream America is, or at least where they were at the time when that episode was released decades ago. Today, the most commonly held notion of a vegan is a person that doesn't consume any animal products - no meat, eggs, or dairy. Although true, the definition falls short. A vegan is someone that has made a pledge, promise, or choice to live a life entirely free from the use of animal products. Or any product that uses animal products in its manufacture or is in any way involved in the harm of animals.

Being a true vegan is no joke. It's a deep conviction, and it's honestly a tough life to live in my opinion. It's a political and almost religious choice, and I have the utmost respect for anyone that truly walks this path (as long as they don't yell at me for eating something with honey in it). You might gather by that admission that I am not a vegan. I am guessing that like me, you may also have experienced a small measure of wrath from a "capital V," vegan at some point in your life. So, let me apologize on behalf of us rational non-animal eaters. Let me get back to the point before I offend my many amazing vegan friends.

As I said, becoming vegan is a huge ethical and philosophical paradigm shift, but becoming *plant-based* is something a little more practical. Something that has interwoven into it a compassionate, environmentally smart, and ethical undertone, but is not derived from those things directly. Instead, the motivation to eat from a plant-based menu usually manifests from a simple desire to be healthier. To mitigate the effects of aging, to have more energy, and to ward off the chances of being ravished with so many of the medical problems that come as a result of our nutritional practices today.

In case you didn't know, WFPB diets *are* directly linked to lower instances of heart disease, diabetes, and cancer. On balance, people who follow a WFPB diet are less fat, less depressed, and more physically active. If you want to take me to task on a couple of those ideas, that means you are already fighting me. So, relax and just be open-minded for now.

So, in summary, you do not have to buy Birkenstocks to complete this program. You do not *ever* have to say, "meat is murder," and you honestly don't even have to adopt the plant-based diet moving forward. But if you are going to put me in charge of your chances for success, you need to trust me and be willing to try new things - even if those new things have your old superstitions tied to them.

For you to be successful in this program, I have only thirty days or so to get your body to stop doing what it is doing now - storing fat and craving sugar - and to *start* doing what we want it to - burn fat, and crave healthy and biochemically rich foods. There is no way I know of to take you that distance while you are holding on to old paradigms and putting old familiar poisons into your body. Remember, your body is not just bloated - it's broken.

David Clark

Just like we have been doing since the dawn of civilization, we are going to use plants to heal us.

"But where do you get your protein?" This is the Holy Grail of questions in the vegan universe. The question that any veggie-muncher answers all day, every day. The outlandish truth is that a person that follows a WFPB diet will typically get *more* protein than a person on the standard American diet. Yes, you read that right. Yes, you should read it again.

If you are already following a plant-based diet, you can probably skip this next paragraph or two, as you've likely heard all this before, but if you are brand new to the idea of getting protein from plants, I am going to point you in two directions. One - The gorilla. You know. Chimps, Great Apes, Bonobos. Our closest related living ancestors who, by the way, manage to be very strong without eating any meat at all. Still, think vegetarians are weak? Two - The movie *Game Changers*. If you want to geek out on the science behind the plant-based diet complete with graphics, studies, and interviews from world-class doctors, researchers, and athletes, you will find the movie full of information to digest (pun intended). But in case you've never heard of Netflix, or don't like documentaries, I will go over the basics here for the benefit of those that haven't heard the protein argument before.

First off, humans don't need protein - we *make* protein. Humans do not need to eat complete chains of protein in the form of muscle from other animals. Instead, we make protein chains internally.

Our bodies are basically in the protein production business. Like almost all mammals, we get the building blocks for our protein from plants. Protein is comprised of chains of amino acids that our bodies need for tissue repair, cellular function, and of course, to make muscle. Our bodies make many of the amino acids necessary for this at a cellular level. The amino acids that we don't make internally are called *essential amino acids* and need to be provided to us through dietary consumption. This might be hard to believe… but yes, *all* the essential amino acids we need are found in plants.

You don't need to go out and find an excessively large variety of various plants to get what you need. You don't need to combine foods together, you just need to "eat your veggies" as mom said, and you will get protein in abundance. Yes, actually, you will not only get a *sufficient* amount of protein, you'll likely get a *surplus*. Studies show that plant-based eaters on balance get more protein than meat-eaters. I would say it again, but you probably reread it on your own. The old, antiquated idea that we need to eat muscle to make muscle is almost as scientific as saying you should eat hair if bald, or that eating bones will make you taller.

Something worth mentioning is that even at this time, when this plant-based research is finally being shared on a global platform, the topic remains controversial. The *science* isn't controversial, but the topic itself is. For some reason, the belief that we don't need to eat meat to live touches us in a deep and

David Clark

personal way. It hits on our childhood, what our parents told us, and of course all those paid-for endorsements by doctors. All deeply rooted in our young, developing minds and reinforced on every television show, movie, book, or advertisement you have ever seen. You have perhaps a million reference points in your mind that cry out in protest when the idea that eating meat is unhealthy rears its ugly head. Combine that with the picture that most people have of the vegetarian lifestyle - also reinforced negatively in media - and you have one big gnarly paradigm to overcome.

But we know now that we don't need to eat meat to live, or to be strong - that is irrefutable. We can simply point to the numerous examples of world-class athletes, bodybuilders, strong men and women, and everyday people who are thriving on a plant-based diet to see it's possible. Did you know that a couple of years ago, we had a vegan as "The World's Strongest Man?" So even if I can't persuade you that being a plant-based athlete is optimal, it should not be too difficult for you to believe that you can at least do this program and be quite confident you won't die. After all, I started a thirty-day vegan challenge ten years ago and never looked back, and I've run over one-hundred footraces and managed to go from confirmed fat ass to endurance badass while eating nothing but plants. Did you hear that mic-drop?

"I didn't climb my way to the top of the food chain to eat grass." I don't even need a dime for every time I have heard that statement - I might be rich if I had a dime for every time I've *said* it *myself.* It showcases another deep misunderstanding of who we are as a species. For the record, it should be glaringly obvious that we are most certainly not on the top of the food chain… Wander into the wild for a few days, and it will become abundantly clear where you stand. But that point aside, it might come as a huge shock to many people (it did to me) that we as humans are not carnivores, nor did we evolve from carnivores.

As predators, humans are actually dogshit. We are not fast. We are not particularly strong. We do not possess the required sharp teeth to rip flesh from bone, and we don't have the stomach acid content to break down uncooked flesh. Before you point to those tiny little baby canines in your mouth, just remember that big strong gorilla ancestor of yours? Yeah, well, his sharp teeth are there merely to scare off competitors, not to eat other animals - you can also thank him for all those wide flat teeth that herbivores have to gnash nuts, berries, and plants. I have just one last point - we don't have a short intestinal tract as carnivores do, humans have long intestines to digest the nutrients from plants slowly. When we eat meat, it sits and rots inside us for days until we can finally push it out.

That ugly business aside, I will very willingly say that humans are omnivores of a sort. We aren't omnivores in the sense of bears or dogs, animals that can truly eat and efficiently process both raw meat and plants, but we are omnivores in the sense that the human species is nature's ultimate survival machine.

David Clark

In this area, we are most certainly at the top of the chain. No other species can do what we do. We can live in extreme cold or extreme heat. We can live on mountain tops or in the desert. Yes, we can *survive* on meat or plants. We can survive on tree bark and berries if need be. We won't achieve supreme health or optimal performance like this, but when it comes to survival - we are the "New York Yankees" of all animals.

But you aren't trying to simply survive this rehab. What we are looking for is what is *optimal* and what will give us the greatest potential to heal and what will produce the best internal environment for us to restore balance to all of our hormonal, endocrinal, and metabolic functions. We want to take all the poisons out of our bodies so that we can take all the poisons out of our minds, and all the destruction out of our habits. For that we need to eat only foods nature has provided for our own unique biology.

I am not going to attempt to cover the topic of factory farming, how corrupt and poisonous the animal food chain has become, or the environmental disaster that is animal agriculture. It is beyond the scope of this book, and I am not on a mission to change your politics. For now, I am just on a mission to change your life. But I will say that we are very far removed even from our most recent ancestors (grandma and grandpa) who ate animals, too. Today we are eating animals that are grown solely to be food. Today's meat comes from chemically altered, steroid injected and disease-prone livestock, not from wild animals. If you do want to learn about factory farming and how it affects us all, watch the documentary "Cowspiracy."

Aside from allowing your body to heal itself, let me talk a little about why a plant-based diet will help you lose weight. As discussed in chapter two, what we eat has a profound effect on not just how we store fat, but what we desire to eat. Processed foods like dairy and sugar and highly saturated fats from animal products affect the brain's chemistry as well as our metabolic function. By consuming only WFPB calories, we will be effectively stopping the endless craving and fat storage cycle. Just like the alcoholic, so too must we go "cold turkey" (terrible analogy). We have to stop, at a cellular level, the constant craving, and hunger that is produced from bombarding our nutrient delivery system with items that affect us more like drugs.

One last food-drug comparison - when we ingest a narcotic painkiller such a Percocet into our bodies, it is introduced via our digestive tract. It possesses no nutritional benefit, has no calories, and will not sustain us in any way. Instead, what happens is this powerful substance passes the blood-brain barrier and produces a profound impact on neurological function and perception.

Similarly, when foreign or highly processed "foods" enter our digestive tract, the body is unsure how to process them. The initial elation from junk food creates a false sense of benefit, and the experience gets stored as a pleasurable experience causing undesirable and disastrous effects on our behavior. These "food-drugs" cause us to start pleasure-seeking, and we begin losing track of the long-term consequences in favor of the immediate effect. This makes weight-loss an almost impossible task. Our bodies and minds are virtually at war with each other, and we are caught in the crossfire. Therefore, we must eliminate *anything* that will make us fall prey to the emotional and behavioral pull of catastrophic calories while we are trying to establish a whole new mind-body universe. Imagine if while trying to establish a meditation practice, you played Slayer in your Air Pods at full volume… I've tried, it doesn't work.

If you are worried about carbs, I feel you. It's scary to think of eating carbs, especially if, like me, you have previously lost weight on a high protein or zero-carb diet. So, you know, you don't really *need* to eat a ton of carbs on a plant-based diet if you don't want to. While trying to lose weight, I recommend you don't eat any fruit. Not because fruit is bad for you - it isn't. But because fruit is nature's fuel. Right now, you probably have a very abundant fuel supply saved up for a rainy day. So, let's grab that fuel off the hips before we stop at Citgo. But while you are contemplating your past diet choices, remember that the low-carb diet ultimately failed you. It didn't work. Otherwise, you would have stayed with it. We need to make sure the impact extends past the end of the **Radical Rehab**. It needs to have a lasting effect on how you think, how you feel, and how your body functions. The WFPB diet is completely aligned with the goal of repairing your sluggish metabolism and rebalancing your endocrine function.

The last part of why a WFPB diet is such an important part of this program is harder to quantify. It's spiritual. When I first switched to eating plants, I would have never thought it would have an impact on my spiritual health, but it did, eventually. There is some deeply hidden karmic barometer in the human soul that is inactive during conflict. I suspect we know deep inside our relationship with food and animals is wrong. Even if you disagree with me and feel that it is moral and justified to eat an animal (and I won't argue with you), we know that the casual way we take life in today's world is disconnected at best, and morally reprehensible at worst.

We are a universe away from respectfully taking an animal's life for survival compared to walking through a grocery store with thirty-five different kinds of hot dogs. Going plant-based for these thirty days will connect you to what you eat. It will temporarily disconnect you from the cycle of runaway animal destruction that is today's factory farming. Most importantly, it will provide you with an unexpected spiritual connection to the world. Even if you go back to a diet with meat in it, you will be more connected, more mindful, and more present in your actions and choices, and that is exactly how you will beat this addiction cycle forever.

David Clark

Chapter 6
The Ultimate Machine

"If you hear a voice within you say, 'you cannot paint,' then by all means paint and that voice will be silenced."
— Vincent Van Gogh

In the *Bhagavad Gita*, the ancient warrior text about Prince Arjuna and his spirit guide, Lord Krishna, we see a picture of a *complete* warrior-being. It's not just a deep devotion to meditation, not just a righteous practice of living, but also a strong physical body that makes Prince Arjuna the complete warrior. He is the embodiment of all human strength in one person. This isn't exactly what might be presented as a *warrior* in America today, though.

In most popular movies and books, we usually place the spiritual warrior in a weak, frail, or aging body - Yoda comes to mind from "Star Wars" or The Oracle from "The Matrix." When we see the *complete* warrior, it is most often represented as a team or collaboration of warriors, each displaying mastery in one focus. The brawny muscle-clad gladiator, fighting alongside the crafty intelligent, but wispy elf, and of course, the spiritual wizard, barely able to walk without his staff, but can vanquish the enemy with the magic of the universe.

This notion in western society that the mind, body, and spirit are three separate entities is pervasive. Without knowing it, we subconsciously parse this disjointed picture of humanity throughout society as if one particular person might possess a strong body yet have a weak mind. Someone else may have a strong spiritual nature but a fragile body, etc. But we are *all* capable of developing and even mastering physical, intellectual, and spiritual prowess. I will further submit that it is a complete illusion to suggest that we could somehow develop mastery in one of these areas while ignoring the others. Or worse, only be bestowed the potential for excellence in one.

We may identify someone as strong in one realm and weak in another, but when we become devoted to a complete mastery of self, every part of the whole needs to grow in response. Certainly, we are not all going to be six feet tall, and three-hundred pounds of muscle, and not all of us are going to be Albert Einstein. But physical strength can manifest itself in everybody. We can *all* develop our minds, increase our cognition, and we can all draw from the power of the universe too. This is an important concept to understand. Because you can never achieve a healthy and fit body while you are poisoning it at the same time. You can never achieve a calm internal state while your body is dying a slow, sedentary death. You can never truly establish a deep spiritual connection to the universe while taking actions that harm others. We either grow as a whole entity, or we are just borrowing from one account to grow the other.

David Clark

Over the course of the next thirty days, you are going to heal your broken mind by establishing a new connection to what you eat. You are going to tend to the spiritual pain you have accumulated in your past through meditation, and you are also going to rebuild the temple that is your physical body. So, get ready, because you're going to become a warrior - or *athlete* - if you prefer. This, as is all the tenets of the rehab program, is non-negotiable. You must be willing to develop your physical body. You must become willing to work hard, learn to handle pain, and develop a relationship with being uncomfortable. Not only will becoming an athlete give you the physical changes you desire, a higher metabolism, more muscle, and less fat, it will also give you a focus and purpose that will touch your evolutionary spirit.

Being a physical being is hardwired into our DNA. For our ancestors, merely surviving a single day was a massive accomplishment that required a high level of physicality. In today's world of comfort and anchored inertia, we are missing out on the very part of what connects us to our evolutionary spirit. In other words, we are incomplete and unfulfilled without some level of sweat and blood. When our bodies are fit, everything that we do is enhanced. We think better, we make smarter choices, we handle stress better, and we experience the world more vividly.

Imagine your current body as the old black and white television console your grandparents used to have in the living room. You remember the one, right? With the record player on top and speakers the size of mini-fridges covered in wicker. Today, as you play your life channel, you are getting old analog sound, with blurry and distorted images on a heavy glass screen, and you only have three channels to choose from - not too exciting, is it? At the end of this rehab, I want your body to go from 1980 to 2020. When you are fit and functioning, you will be a "4k" High-Definition Smart Television with a Bose Soundbar. In your "new life" movie, you will be able to see miles into the background of three-dimensional landscapes, you will make out the threads in the lumberjack's flannel shirt, and the explosions will send bass that hits you in the chest like a heavy punching bag. Your fit body will not just make you look and feel better. It will allow you to experience life on an exponentially exaggerated plane.

Question. Has it ever struck you as odd that we even need gyms and health clubs? Imagine an average day for a human just a few generations ago. Hard work, physical activity, and stressing the body was a part of almost every task. We fixed our cars, lifted and chopped wood, walked to the other side of town, built and repaired houses - and that's just modern man. Never mind the hunting, fishing, and farming that was requisite for our postmodern relatives.

In today's world, our bodies are so atrophied from their incapacity, that we have invented treadmills to run on and step mills to mimic climbing stairs. We go to fancy clubs and lift heavy objects to grow our muscles, and then we post to Instagram so our sedentary friends can tell us how amazing we are… Amazing compared to *what*? The point is we were made to move. It's how we heal, how we grow, and how we find wellbeing and a sense of accomplishment. I hate to break this to you, but I bet you could use more pain in your life. The world has become a great big race to see who can invent an easier way to live and experience life. All the while our souls are dying along with our lower backs.

In the **Radical Rehab** program**,** I want you to challenge yourself physically. Sorry, but you need to experience pain so that you can grow stronger. You need to develop the inner relationship and mental strength that will allow you to go to the gym and endure workouts so that you have a glorious and solid foundation to build your new life on.

I want you to rekindle the part of you that lays in recess and the warrior spirit in you that is there to fend off invading tribes and climb over mountains to secure new land. Before we are done, you are going to need a big, gnarly, and scary physical goal to help you rise to the challenge.

But chances are, someone has told you that you need to set small incremental goals to be successful. Someone has likely postulated to you that the path of success is laid upon a road built by accomplishing small obtainable goals that will lead to bigger and better breakthroughs. Bullshit. I'll wager you've tried small goals and moderation more times than that critic has opened Facebook.

Those of us that are caught in the web of overeating, addiction, and obesity have tried every diet, every psychological trick, and every ritual out there - twice. We end up flat on our face at Wendy's dipping our French fries into our Frosties. Moderation is for people too afraid to succeed at something big. So how about this? How about you go all-in on something huge? Running a marathon. Climbing a mountain. Doing a triathlon or whatever it is that speaks to you. If nothing is speaking to you, start looking for something that does.

I am someone who has been exactly where you are, afraid to fail and afraid to start, stuck in the concrete, and tired of the relentless nagging thoughts. Feeling the weight of your body that is almost as heavy as the gnawing thoughts that keep biting at the ends of your sofa cushions like an unwelcome mouse. You know the thoughts, right? The ones that ask: Am I doomed to live this life? Is this who I really am? Is there more to life? Am I selling myself short? Let me answer for you - yes. There is more to life. You are definitely selling yourself short, and it should start pissing you off. I've been there, and it sucks ass. I've quit on myself a thousand times until one day I got tired of eating shit. So, think big! You will never know how strong you are until you place yourself in a position where being stronger than you have ever been is required.

But here is the gem that so many people miss when digging for a big goal. We have to dream big. Dream scary, and then put that dream away for a

David Clark

while. We can't try to carry the weight of the goal everywhere we go, or it will fold us up faster than Superman on laundry day. The goal sits off in the distance. It's real. As real as you and me. I want you to visit it regularly. But don't live there.

Don't think of the work we do as the torture needed to get somewhere else. To make the big change, we must surrender to finding joy in the work at hand. I've run one-hundred miles over thirty times, and yet if I let the magnitude of running non-stop for seventeen to twenty hours sit on my brain too long, it will crush me. At the starting line of a one-hundred-mile run, I must commit to the race, but then never even consider the finish line until it springs up from the ground in front of me. I run one mile at a time, embracing the struggle, joyful through the journey, and committed to the end. That's how I did weight-loss too. That's exactly how I want you to approach your new life.

So, now I ask you before you start your **Radical Rehab** - is this new life real, or is it a fucking wish? If you want it to be real, you have to commit to doing the work of that day. You don't analyze it or question it. You go to work. Run the mile you're on. Do that, and I promise you will make it. Execute this plan flawlessly, and you'll get the results you want. Fuck around, and you might make it – and you might not. But know this - my money is on you. I believe in you. I don't think you made it all the way here just to give up. After all, if you were going to quit, you would have done it by now.

One *final note before you start the* **Radical Rehab** *program: If you choose to read the entire program before you begin, that's fine. I highly recommended it. But when you are ready, make sure you start this program with an open mind and an open schedule. Meaning, do not start if you know you have a wedding coming up, or a vacation, or if anything is impending that you know will knock you off course. Once you start, you need to be committed to seeing this all the way through.*

Lastly, no drugs or alcohol of any kind in any amount (medications excluded) during the program. I do have to remind you that before you start any workout program that it's a good idea to go to your doctor and make sure you have medical clearance to start.

David Clark

STAGE 1

Chapter 7
Unfuck Your Fridge

"Rock bottom became the solid foundation on which I rebuilt my life."
— *J.K. Rowling*

You are done eating shit in your life. You know that today's processed foods send you into a pleasure-seeking loop that will ultimately spiral you to an early death. You know that your body has been taken hostage by unnatural levels of salt, fat, and sugar, and has been forced into becoming a fat-seeking missile. You have seen a glimpse of how your own ideas of food and comfort have all conspired to make you miserable. Finally, the work to fill this sinkhole is at hand.

If you are not ready to go to war now, you should be. Now is not the time to show fear or to be tentative. This is the time for you to step up to the challenge of your life. There is a stronger, more confident person within, and that person needs to be in charge now. So, go watch Rocky, crank up the Slayer, go run around the block, do some pushups or whatever you have to do to psych yourself up. Once you are ready to run through a brick wall, come back and dive back in.

We are finally here - day one of rehab. The foundation of this program rests in taking ten massive steps I call **Radical Rehab.** The program is designed to completely destroy the comfortable prison you've built around your life. The **Radical Rehab** and its steps are going to help you shatter the reflection you see in the mirror. The steps are going to help you expose all the lies you've been telling yourself, face the fears you've buried deeply in your heart, and finally set in place a new paradigm that allows you to live free from the demons that cause you to overeat. You are going to reset your body, heal your broken and malfunctioning systems, and build yourself a life so amazing that you'll wonder why you ever lived the way you do now. But you didn't think you'd be able to do all that without getting your hands dirty, did you?

Of course, you didn't. So, it shouldn't come as a shock that I have some chores for you to do. Just like Ralph Macchio had to suck it up in "The Karate Kid" and paint Mr. Miyagi's fence and sand the floor to learn karate, you are going to have to trust me that there is a hidden purpose for all that I ask you to do. Grab some gloves, some spray cleaner, and some heavy-duty trash bags because the very first thing we are going to do is get your kitchen in order. That's right - shit is getting real.

"The kitchen is the heart of the home," they say. Well, it is also the heart of your health. Everything you bring into your kitchen eventually goes into your mouth and therefore into your blood, which pumps through your heart. It's about time we started respecting your refrigerator for what it is. It is not just a box to keep your drinks cold and your food from spoiling. It's the epicenter for all the nutrition that every person in your house receives, and there is nothing in your life with greater influence over what you eat than your fridge. That might sound like an overstatement, but it isn't. You might say that certainly your cravings, your habits, and work life have greater impact over what you eat than your refrigerator, but if you dig deeper, you'll find that's not so. How you treat your fridge effects how you think at work, your state of mind when you get to work, and what you eat when you get home.

I will submit that how you do even the smallest thing in your life is how you do the biggest things - there is behavioral precedent for all your actions. We like to separate or compartmentalize things, but the reality is all that we do is tied to all that we think. If we are willing to pick up junk at the grocery store, carry it to our cars, take it to our house and place it the fridge, what are the chances you will abstain from the lure of breakroom donuts? And conversely, if your entire fridge is habitually stocked with only healthy and vibrant eats, you are less likely to indulge in something that you know will make you feel like crap. Let that sink in. While it does, let's get back to your kitchen so I can show you how cleaning out your fridge is also a way to clean out your head.

You can't finish a race without getting to the starting line. If I told you that the Boston Marathon covers the road from Hopkinton to Boston and is 26.2 miles long, that gives you a general picture of the race. But if your goal was to actually compete in the Boston Marathon, you would need much more information. You would need to know *exactly* when and where the race starts, for example. Not only would you need this to comply with the rules, but your *mind* would need to know the specific details so it could arrange the internal resources to complete the goal.

You couldn't just wake up on Patriots' Day and immediately start running a marathon from bed. Imagine if your brain was running the marathon as you left the hotel, jumped on the shuttle, and stood around for hours in the runners' village, the whole time your feet marching up and down on their own with your brain going non-stop already internally running the roads, the turns, the mile splits, considering the crowds, the other runners, and the weather. Your heart rate would be elevated, and your adrenaline would be flowing while you just stood in place... By the time the actual race started you would be mentally exhausted and likely drop out by the first "5k."

Our minds need specific details to be able to allocate mental focus and resources for any large undertaking. Yet, many times we start large projects on little more than a general notion of what we want or hope to do. We wake up and proclaim that we are *going vegan* or starting a gym program or losing one-hundred pounds - all with no clear and specific break from our regularly scheduled internal environment - and that's the reason we fail.

Your mind can't accomplish much with the command "I want to eat healthy today." It's wishy-washy and it's muddled. But if you say, "I am going to eat fruit for breakfast, a spinach salad for lunch, and sweet potato tacos for dinner," the mind has a very clear target. Your chances for success are greatly enhanced because there is an overriding and clear directive.

Whenever we are to accomplish something *big,* there has to a be a *big* break from the norm. We have to create the internal space for new behaviors and actions. That is what unfucking your fridge is about. It's a ritualistic dance, it's a pilgrimage or rite of passage to signify to your mind that you are going in a brand-new direction. We have to take an action that sends a clear message that the old way is over, and that the new way is starting.

But humans are programmed to hold on. We cling to the familiar. We resist the new. We don't like the idea of clearing out our comfortable illusions in favor of the unknown. We are like the person trying to get the groceries to the house from the car in one trip. We are loaded from armpits to forearms with grocery bags. A bag looped over each finger, walking sideways, spread-legged, head cocked to the side. Like a deranged spider-mom trying desperately not to drop any of the precious cargo.

This act of cleaning out the fridge is not just a chance to clear out the old way, it is a meditation, too.

It's a chance for your body, mind, and spirit to work together. This process will be a choice that starts in your mind, requires your body to act, and has direct impact on your spiritual identity. But aren't I just cleaning the fridge you ask? No. Fuck no. You are cleansing your house and your entire being in the process. I need you to be aware of that as you go about this task. But, yeah… it's also about getting those Oreos and frozen waffles into the trash, where they belong.

One of the reasons alcoholics must hit rock bottom before they stop drinking, is so the consequences of their actions become painful enough to warrant change. But there is another bigger purpose for rock bottom - so there is a clear break in the old narrative. We have to interrupt the signal we are getting from our subconscious mind. Our inner voices have become very adept at moving us along the conveyor line of terrible consequences. We forgive junk food (or alcohol) for all the terrible things it is doing to us until one day we realize that we are in an abusive relationship. We are getting the shit beat out of us at home and telling everyone at work that we fell down the stairs.

Rock bottom is when "it could always be worse" is no longer powerful enough to keep us captive. It's when it becomes time to pack our bags and get the fuck out. But to find the strength to walk away from a bad relationship, we need something out of the ordinary to happen. Something that breaks the cycle and lets us start to see things in a new way. It's

David Clark

not just the fear of losing their house or pending legal repercussions that makes an addict move forward. Something has to happen internally to wake them up to what's happening.

We are going to go deep on this in steps four through six, but for now it's important to understand that we are going to light some shit on fire. We need those smoke detectors to go off. Just like a forest fire, it will eventually create a nutrient-rich substrate for new and unimaginable growth. We need a little kitchen fire to clear the way for you to grow. But for the record, DO NOT SET FIRE TO YOUR KITCHEN. I was being metaphorical… strange times we live in.

This **Radical Rehab** includes taking **ten** major life-altering **steps**. It will be very straightforward and clear how to follow the plan as you go, but just so you know, underneath each of these steps are numbered **intentions** that should be done before moving on to the following step. Think of the steps themselves as the lesson, and the **intentions** as the homework. These expansions are designed to make sure that you have clearly internalized the concept and applied it to yourself before you move on. The **intentions** will help you dig deep and have a more expanded experience during your rehab. I hope you can resist the temptation to do only the steps without completing the **intentions**, but if for some reason you do, make sure you come back to this book for the mastery **intentions** at a later date.

Each section of the **Radical Rehab** also includes **meditation**, **action** (physical movement), and **nutritional inspiration** (a nutritious whole-food, plant-based recipe idea). Some of the steps will have large-scale physical tasks that will take much effort, and other steps will seem milder by contrast, but each step is a specific brick needed to build a very specific structure. Just like when I am designing a complex training plan for a competitive athlete, the entire program is progressive. Each workout, rest day, and week is all tied into a predetermined outcome - so are the sessions you will be undertaking.

Some of you reading this book are already athletes or gym rats. If you are, I want you to challenge yourself to expand your training with a renewed purpose and intensity. You can, of course, simply maintain your current level of training if that's all you can wrap your mind around. The important thing is that you *keep training* through all the ups and downs of the rehab.

For those who are not currently in a fitness program, I did include some basic suggestions listed as **actions**, for you. Make sure you do them. Hopefully I have made the case for how important it is that you start treating your body like a machine. We are going to drive that machine home in steps seven through nine, so get the engine running now with these daily actions.

As for **meditations** I've included, they are not merely inspirational quotes, they are deep thoughts that I want you to explore. Write about them in your journal - yes, you are going to be keeping a journal - and meditate on them as well. Since I can't get you up and doing everything on day one, I will start to implement the journal and meditation within the first few days of the program. For now, just know that these are important and should be explored from day one going forward.

The **nutritional inspirations** are just that - some of my own recipes that may serve as inspiration for you to create some of your own amazing plant-based meals. I've shied away from including a detailed meal plan in these sections, not just because it's impossible to create one plan that will be appealing for everyone, but because I want you to do some work on your own. The work itself has value and I want you to embrace plant-based cooking. I want you to be inspired to re-engineer your current favorite meals into healthier options. I want you to investigate and find what works inside your own mind and what appeals to your personal cravings.

I realize that not everyone works the same schedule and that is why I have resisted the urge to create a rigid calendar with this plan. Not everyone has the flexibility to execute a rehab program in the exact manner that I designed it. So instead, I have broken the program into the **ten steps** that lay before you. These steps are proven to get you where you want to be. They are the result not just of my own transformation, but an accumulation of the hundreds of clients I have worked with personally as well as concepts from the best of the worlds of addiction recovery, professional coaching, professional athletics, business leadership, and of course spiritual revolutionaries such as the Buddha. Please take the program seriously.

A note of caution for my "type As" out there... you cannot "race" this program. You cannot move on to step two until you are firmly standing on step one. You cannot get to the top of this climb unless you take each step in the order prescribed. In other words, you must start on step one and complete each step, in order. Don't make this a checklist - experience it as it's written. That said, how much time you spend in-between the steps is up to you. You have *some* flexibility, but it is paramount that you never lose connection to the process. You cannot do steps one through five, then go on vacation and expect to jump into step six when you return. Do not rush through either. This is not a ten-day program. You will need a period of time (I would say somewhere close to thirty days) where this program is the single-most important thing in your life.

RADICAL REHAB

STEP ONE

"I promised myself I was done eating shit and acted on this declaration by unfucking my fridge."

We start step one with a promise and a complete refrigerator purge. The promise is to yourself - and it's to be made out loud. Look into the mirror and say, "I'm done eating shit" and mean it - literally and figuratively. You are done poisoning your body with a diet comprised mostly of junk and toxic food-like products. You are also done eating shit in the form of negative self-talk. Starting today, you are leaving the old behind, and only looking ahead to wherever this journey takes you.

With that promise made, you will act on this declaration by unfucking your fridge. So, take everything out of your fridge and place it on the floor or counter. Do not half-ass this - do not do a modified version. If for some reason, you can't get enough leverage on yourself to take this action completely as directed, then you have nothing - it's the first step for crying out loud. If you are resisting, ask yourself why you aren't willing to take the first step. If you still can't get yourself to act, you might as well put the book down and head to the nearest burger joint - game over. I don't mean to start off so aggressively, but there will undoubtedly be people that will read right past this step and think, "My fridge is good. Next!" Don't be that person.

So, when I say take everything out of your fridge, I mean *everything*. Every condiment, box of baking soda, unidentified Tupperware container, and even all the shelves and drawers. Yes, take out the crisper and every railing or divider that can be removed without a tool (don't forget the freezer, too). While you are doing this, I want you to think about *why* you are doing it. What chain of events led you here? What were the lowest moments of your overeating career? Really connect with how you have interacted with food throughout your life. Then take pride in the fact that you are taking responsibility for it now.

Try to make an emotional connection or attach a specific memory to every item you take out of the fridge. Once you are staring at an empty white box, take a look at the condition of the fridge. Is it messy? Were there spoiled items in there? How does it smell? Over the years, was the fridge a place that you brought clean, living, and vibrant food to feed yourself and your family? Or was it a collection receptacle for rotting flesh and mood-altering drugs pretending to be food? There is no right or wrong answer. I only want you to be present with the role your fridge has played in your life. When you are done, look around at all the food, packages, jars, bags, and containers on your floor and counters. Take pictures of it all. Then throw it all away. Every item -

David Clark

no matter how recently purchased, no matter how likely you are to reuse it later. I need you to draw a line in the sand and fucking throw it all in the dumpster.

There are a couple of exceptions from the throwaway list: any whole fresh fruit or vegetable may be saved, and any bottled water or fresh non-dairy milk, such as almond milk, cashew milk, etc. can be kept. For the next thirty days, nothing will be placed into the fridge that isn't a WFPB item. But don't freak out just yet. Before you start imagining a life without cow's milk or steak, I want to remind you this is a finite program with a beginning and an end. The intent here is to not just to break the cycle of addictive behaviors, but also to heal your broken body, and the whole-food plant-based items will do just that. You don't have to commit to anything outside of thirty days for now, but remember, you promised me full commitment until then.

Before you place anything in that disgusting fridge, we have some cleaning to do. Time to have at it with the cleaner. Last time I did this (and I still do it once a year), I sprayed the fridge down with cleaner and used paper towels to scrub down the sides. The bottom and sides of the fridge had a syrupy, thick, and hardened goop from some spilled item long forgotten, so I had to pour boiling hot water over it. That seemed to do the trick, and it broke up easily, and I mopped out the fridge floor with some heavy bath towels.

Do whatever you have to do - be like Vincent from "Pulp Fiction" and "clean up the brain pieces." But instead of cleaning the back seat of the getaway car, your job is to make that fridge shine. "The Wolf" is coming to inspect your work, so raise your standards to the highest level possible and make sure every square inch of that fridge is clean. If you've never seen "Pulp Fiction," and have no clue what I am talking about, just clean that fridge!

Once again, take the time to connect to why you are doing this. Pay attention to your breathing; think about how good it feels to be getting your house in order. Get excited about what is happening. Take the shelves and drawers and soak them in hot soapy water and give them a thorough cleaning too.

Okay. So, you've thrown away all that junk. You've cleaned the appliance inside and out, and you've placed the clean shelves and drawers back in. But there's more bad news… you have to repeat this process for the pantry. Get rid of all those crackers, cookies, snacks, and junk items and clean off those shelves, too. Now take some more pictures and take some pride in what you just did. It's no small feat. These actions can have lasting and major repercussions on your whole life moving forward. I cannot overstate this fact. You just interrupted a long continuous chain of bad karma and connected yourself to your food in a way you never have before.

Let's talk about the times you've tried to break your food addiction previously. Why did you fail? Certainly, this isn't the first time you've tried to break the cycle. My guess is you've never been able to get the required leverage on yourself to stick with it for the long haul. Eventually, you self-destructed and ended up in a pizza, ice cream, depression ménage-a-trois, didn't you? Me, too. So, I am going to give you the leverage you need to make it this time - ready? If you don't do this, you will *die*.

How's that sound? If you dismissed that without a thought, stop and think about it for a second. Do you know how fast life can turn on you? Have you seen what happens to a family when the unthinkable happens? When a single visit to the doctor changes every conversation from that moment on? I have. I have listened to a doctor speak nightmarish words to my own father. "It's time to get your affairs in order."

My dad was seventy-two when he heard those words. He wasn't overweight, but he spent his entire life eating without any regard for the difference between food and comfort. I tried to get him to change his diet, even while he was in hospice care, but there is one inescapable fact of life - no one can change another person. If we wait too long, sometimes we can't even save ourselves. My dad did finally resolve himself to change, but for him (and us), it was too late. My dad passed away as I was writing this book.

The point is we need to get leverage on ourselves because the outside stimulus has little effect on us, as my dad's journey shows. But it's important to know that he is not a unique case. Most people will not change how they eat, no matter what health consequences they face. It shows how stubborn we humans truly are. We won't change even when facing death. We dig in because we feel like we are being forced to change, and no one wants to be told what to do. Have you ever refused to do something you actually *wanted* to do, just because someone told you that you should do it? Of course, you have. Even when something as scary as an early death hits us with the need for a diet change, we just do not accept the threat as real. We justify it. We twist the choice around to make sure we don't believe it's real. We stay stuck, stubborn, and dying. That's why it is so important for you to *choose* this now, for yourself *and* your family.

I used to say that if my lifestyle took five years from my life - so be it. In the depths of my addictions, I frequently offered up that I'd rather lose that five years than quit drinking or going to McDonald's. But those aren't real choices. Those choices are being informed by a sick and twisted mind. A healthy mind wouldn't make that call - *ever*. Five fucking years is an eternity when you're "Googling" what it costs to have your father cremated.

I want you to remember this… *Yes or no*. That is your leverage. Every time you think you might drop out of **Radical Rehab** and go back to your old ways - *Yes or no?* Am I giving up on the idea that I can be healthy and happy? *Yes or no?* DO I want to die young? If it's no - keep going. If it's yes - do one-hundred jumping jacks and ask the question again. If it's still no, do twenty-five burpees and ask one more time. If it's still no, run a mile or keep running until you are back in.

So, I challenge you to be mindful of your life and death during your transformation. Attach it to your food. Understand that if you don't do this now, you might never do it. If you *won't* do it now - when will you? You've purchased this book; you are motivated to change right now… why not make *this* the time you do it? If the prospect of cleaning out your fridge is too big for you - you'll never make it. You have to follow through and take the first step even if for no other reason than you are here now, and it's about time you started to believe in yourself and do the things you don't want to do.

At the risk of sounding like your mom – there will be no eating in front of the television during this program either. Instead, your new entertainment is to take in as much information as possible about your eating experience. We need to start connecting your mind to your mouth. I want you to chew slowly (this actually has a profound physical change on digestion). Taste everything you can. Eat as if you have never done it before. Like I mentioned earlier, I want you to be so connected to what you're eating that you feel as if you may have never done it before. Feel the weight of the fork in your hand. Feel what muscles are needed to move that fork to your mouth. Take in the temperature of the food, and the taste of every spice. Feel your feet on the ground as you chew. Think of how your body will use the food to nourish your body. There are thousands of scientific studies that show how mindfulness actually changes biology. Our cells actually behave differently, depending on our mental focus. I'm counting on all that to happen for you.

The impact of mindful eating is almost too vast to calculate. Still, I would have you adopt this mindful eating practice if, for no other reason but to override the deep pattern of mindless eating you have so firmly lodged into your neural pathways. Your brain has developed a complex sequence of events that it puts into place whenever you eat. It's emotional, it's physical, and it's spiritual even if you don't realize it. Every time you place food in your mouth, your brain plays an old familiar song inside your head, just like an old nostalgic ballad can bring back a heartbreak so deeply that you feel that ache in your gut and the tears on your cheeks. You also lose yourself in the soundtrack of your eating habits.

When we aren't present for our meals, we get lost in old sensory experiences that have almost nothing to do with nourishing our bodies and have everything to do with pleasuring ourselves. Time to erase the old playlist from your iPod. You can download a whole new set of kickass music to attach to how you eat. Eventually, you'll find that old band sucked - It was Creed, or possibly Coldplay - yuck.

David Clark

Intention 1

Since you will be planting a spiritual tree that will hopefully grow into a lifelong mediation practice, let's find a place to drop roots. Let's walk the house, visit all the long-forgotten crevasses and closets and mark the spot to set up your mediation basecamp. If you have a den, office, or spare room where you can meditate, that's great, but even choosing a specific corner of the living room will do. It is less important where you choose to meditate than it is that you have a place picked out. Find yourself a comfortable cushion, figure out how to use the timer on your phone, and if you want to go "gangsta level" meditator, get yourself a Buddha statue and a candle.

Ready to take a little stroll down the echoing hallways of the mind? Okay, let's go. You are going to do five minutes of breathwork, and here is how to do it. Turn off the notifications on your phone and then set a five-minute timer. Sit on your cushion or in a chair if you have back or knee problems that will prevent you from sitting on the floor. Sit with your back straight, and your hands folded neatly in your lap. Do not close your eyes. Instead, relax your gaze into a comfortable but unfocused stare. Like you were trying to find the hidden image in one of those auto stereograms, magic-eye photos.

As your gaze relaxes, take in a slow, long inhale. Breathe in as deeply and slowly as you can through your nose, and just as you reach maximum capacity, slowly exhale through the nose and diaphragm, making a very slight snoring sound as you release the air from your lungs. Focus only on your breath. Try to make each inhale and exhale last five seconds or more. Your mind will wander, but simply bring it back to your breath when it does. Repeat this process, bringing your intention back to your breath over and again for the entire five minutes.

Being aware when your mind wanders is part of meditating. Most people feel like they are failing if the mind wanders, but that is not the case. You are building a practice. We are laying the base for all that is to come. Being aware that your mind is wandering, and then redirecting it is precisely one of the skills we are trying to build.

Congrats on completing your first meditation, you dirty hippie.

Intention 2

Grab a pen and paper or create a new file on your laptop. Today, we are going to start a journal. What you put in it is up to you, but you can start by talking about the process of cleaning out your fridge. What did you experience? What was the most unexpected benefit from the purge? What emotions did you feel? There are no rules to the journal, no template or structure to follow. But try to write about what you experienced. Try to describe it so a stranger would understand not just what you were doing, but how it made you feel. What are your concerns and your hopes?

You will need to unpack how you feel to be able to recreate it in on paper, and that is the greatest benefit of the journal. It will help you process what you are doing. I cannot stress how important this is. Not just the journal itself, but your willingness to do it. The mechanics of doing the things that you previously would have skimmed over is where much of the magic is hidden. Do the work. If you haven't executed the program with a pure and complete intention, stop here. Start over. Give yourself the gift of not going through the motions with this rehab.

MEDITATION

There has been tremendous suffering in your life. You have experienced pain, and you've been hurt. The foods you eat cause your body to malfunction and operate poorly. These destructive foods affect how you think, how you feel, and how you behave. If you continue to eat those foods, your body and mind will continue to deteriorate, and you will have increased suffering in all areas of your life.

ACTION

Walk, run, or cycle. Move your body with intention for at least thirty minutes three to four times per week. Break a sweat. No leisurely strolls at the mall.

NUTRITIONAL INSPIRATION

Simple Bowl #1- One of the cornerstones of building a large WFPB recipe toolbox is to think of designing a bowl using a green, a grain, and a bean. You can use this template in any combination to create a number of different, but delicious choices. Broccoli (green), brown rice (grain), and black beans is one of my favorite combos. If you want to spruce it up, throw in some salsa, some guacamole, and then you'll have a delicious first meal of your rehab journey. Simple, healing, and tasty.

David Clark

STEP TWO

"I'm committed to eating only whole plant-based foods for a minimum of thirty days."

Good news: we are going to the store. Yes, step two includes a shopping trip! But don't get too excited; we aren't going to buy that new wardrobe quite yet. But we are going to restock your fridge with WFPB items. I am not going to tell you exactly what to buy because I have no idea what you like or dislike. However, if you have not read this book in its entirety yet, you should look ahead a few days before you go to the grocery store. Spoiler alert: you are going to be doing a special cleanse diet for five days. But whether you are going to start the five-day cleanse tomorrow or in a few days, there are some staples that you'll need for your fridge. Things like greens, grains, and beans.

Most people freeze in their tracks at the prospect of a vegan or WFPB diet - "But what will I eat?!" I personally love beans and rice. I could live on that shit for ten years. But you might find you prefer asparagus and quinoa, or tofu and broccoli, or any of a thousand possibilities. Or you may have even had a psychological barrier to vegetables (don't worry - this will go away). No matter. Rest assured, you are going to learn to think of food and meal construction in an entirely different way over the next thirty days or so.

You'll do well to imagine eating plant-based is more about eating like a gorilla than it is about eating like a rabbit. You will be able to have delicious, amazing food. It's not all salad despite what people say. There are also tacos, lasagna, and veggie burgers. As you know, I will be giving you one of my personal favorite recipes at the end of each **Radical Rehab** step, but for now I'm going to offer you up a general template for your grocery shopping consideration. You may choose to use these suggestions or not, but the important thing is that you get a glimpse under the hood of what WFPB eating looks like.

Here is a very simple meal plan that fits into the overall WFPB parameter of the next thirty days.

Breakfast Ideas:

1. Blueberries, almond milk, and granola
2. Steel cut oats with peanut butter and touch of agave
3. Sprouted grain toast and almond butter

Lunch Ideas:

1. Whole wheat tortilla with nut butter
2. Sweet potato tacos with kale and hummus
3. Beans and rice with asparagus

Dinner Ideas:

1. Kale salad with hummus dressing, tofu, cherry tomatoes, and almond slices

2. Portobello mushrooms served with light oil and baked potato topped with
> salsa and guacamole

3. Arugula salad with raspberry vinaigrette dressing, seitan, artichoke hearts,
> and broccoli

I hope this meal plan inspires you try new things and helps you to take some initiative in expanding your plant-based mind. Make sure you hit up Google and search simple WFPB recipes. Also, take a gander at "Forks Over Knives" (the documentary and the website all have a ton of resources) and fall in love with the idea of learning about eating plants. If on the other hand you just want to keep it simple and follow the meal plan above, that works too. I'll let you in on a secret - for the first year of my own weight-loss journey, eighty percent of what I ate was a whole wheat tortilla with peanut butter and banana. If you can take the boredom, simple can be very effective.

Make a grocery list before you go shopping and map out your meals for the next several days before you create the list. Creating the list will not only make your shopping trip more effective, it will also have a carryover effect for when you have to eat on the fly - meaning you'll have some idea on how to throw together a quick WFPB meal.

If you don't plan in advance and instead just go to the store without a list, you'll likely wander about aimlessly looking for things that fit into the program. You will get frustrated and end up leaving with nothing but a head of lettuce and a tomato. A little trick that may help you to create some flashy new meal ideas is to consider the "normal" things you used to eat and just substitute the meat with a veggie. Instead of using beef in tacos think of using sweet potatoes. Instead of a steak, think of a portobello mushroom.

Here's a quick refresher of the major food categories you'll enjoy on a plant-based diet, with examples:

Fruits: any type of fruit including apples, bananas, grapes, strawberries, citrus fruits, etc.

Vegetables: plenty of veggies including peppers, corn, avocados, lettuce, spinach, kale, peas, collards, etc.

Tubers: root vegetables like potatoes, carrots, parsnips, sweet potatoes, beets, etc.

Whole Grains: grains and other starches in their whole form, such as quinoa, brown rice, millet, whole wheat, oats, barley, etc.

Legumes: beans of any kind, lentils, and similar ingredients.

Other: There are plenty of other foods you can also enjoy including nuts, seeds, tofu, tempeh, whole grain flour and breads, and plant-based milks. However, I recommend eating these foods in moderation, because they are more calorie-dense and can contribute to weight gain.

Items that are *not* allowed: soda, diet soda, or anything heavily processed. Basically, if you couldn't make it yourself by combining several single ingredient items in your own kitchen - don't eat it. But the good news if you're a diet soda junkie like I was, you can have as much sparkling water as you like as long as it's all natural. I am personally keeping the Bubly and the Lacroix companies in business these days.

Intention 3

Imagine a professional golfer walking into the tee box to start an eighteen-hole round of golf. Now visualize the golf club face as it makes contact with the golf ball after the golfer unleashes the controlled violence of the perfectly timed swing. Now consider just a one-millimeter difference in the angle of the club face as it makes contact with the ball. It determines whether the ball lands in the center of the fairway two hundred fifty yards away, or whether it goes two hundred fifty yards, to the left and out of bounds. Not only did that single shot take on an entirely different landing point based on a small fraction of deviance, but now the next shot has been altered as well, and in effect the whole round of golf. All due to an infinitesimal angle variance.

With that perspective in mind, give yourself some credit for making a paradigm shift and a major change of course in your life. The trajectory of your earthly journey has diverged, and like that golf ball, where you land now would be impossible to calculate. It might not seem like it but even a small change makes a big difference when you project it out, and your change was not just a small fractional anomaly, no, your action is something bold and explosive. You stepped into the tee box, rotated around to the opposite side of the ball and launched it backward toward the ocean. You are now on a whole new path, in an entirely different game.

To keep the wind in the sails of your new voyage, let's put some intention into your journaling and meditating. Try to quantify how different your daily life has been since you started this rehab. How different do you feel? Can you articulate the new plot of trajectory you are on? Write it all down. Wait until you get it all out before you edit and correct your spelling. Keep the flow of words going. Do not interrupt the connection if you find yourself in the beautiful flow-state of writing. If it's clunky and awkward - that's okay too. Just get it all out onto the paper (or screen). Trust me, we are going somewhere with all this. Nothing in this program is filler.

David Clark

Everything here has a specific purpose.

Your meditation practice today will increase to ten minutes, but the focus and intention will remain the same. Deep inhales. Slow exhales. Relax your gaze, focus on nothing and bring your thoughts back to your breath. Resist the temptation to judge your practice. Do not compare your meditation to something arbitrary and an imaginary picture of what you think it should be. Instead experience it. Allow it to happen on its own with you as the observer.

Intention 4

Let's allow the work we have done to take hold. You have changed your routine quite a bit over the last few days and today is a day to eat clean, healthy foods, to continue to be present in the new heartbeat of your home, and of course, to work on your breathing.

When learning a new skill such as martial arts, playing the piano, or even calculus, it is important to allow the new information that we have absorbed to take root and begin to sprout. As an amateur boxer, I find that after working tirelessly on a new defensive drill or working with a new trainer, a small break in training allows me to return and apply the new skills at a much higher level than if I continued to go through the motions.

With that in mind, I want you to set aside a few moments before you meditate to reflect on the changes you have made. Write it all down in your journal. Mentally revisit all the garbage you pulled from the fridge. Think of the living, brilliant, and energetic food that you brought into it and think of how the food that you are eating is healing you. Think of the gift of life that is incubating in your new body. Afterward, set your timer for ten minutes and focus on your breathing.

MEDITATION

Change is real. Despite what some people may tell you about the impossibility of making a fundamental and permanent change, it happens - and you need to believe in it. The possibility of you making the change you desire rests solely on you buying into the notion that you can do this. You will never be able to ride out the unavoidable low points unless you believe that change is real.

ACTION

Walk, run or cycle. Move your body with intention for at least thirty minutes three to four times per week. Break a sweat, no leisurely strolls at the mall.

NUTRITIONAL INSPIRATION

Easy Spicy Sweet Potato Tacos - Using either sprouted grain tortillas or corn tortillas for the shell, chop some kale, tomato, onion and jalapeño (or

David Clark

habanero for extra spicy) as the toppings. Cut sweet potatoes into French fry shapes and either grill, or air-fry to your desired level of firmness. Spice with salt, pepper, and chipotle seasoning. Place into tortilla shell, add kale, tomato, onion and peppers. Top with guacamole and Sabra Spicy Hummus. Eat that shit up.

STEP THREE

"I completed a five-day healing ritual."

Today will be the start of a five-day healing ritual based on the power of fasting. But don't worry, you are not going to be going five days without eating anything. There is a considerable amount of research that shows fasting has been historically a regular part of human life. It makes sense when you think about it. Our ancestors did not have the benefit of grocery stores, weekly paychecks, or even county jail to ensure that three meals a day would be provided. Sometimes, even with considerable effort to hunt and gather, there was simply no food to be found. What research shows us is that when the body goes into a fasting period, our biological system ups its game in response. The body goes into a sort of spring cleaning of the metabolism - it starts to clear out toxins, reboot sluggish systems, and even increases the production of its own stems cells to heal torn tissues, repair fractured bones, and to replenish previously depleted stem cell stores.

When our bodies acclimate to stress from combat, like running from tigers and moving rocks around the village (or from working out at Lifetime Fitness), part of our autonomic physiological healing process comes from our body's stem cells. The stem cells increase blood flow to the area, reduce inflammation, and act as the general managers of biological repair. These stem cells handle all of the

David Clark

day-to-day repairs our bodies require. Additionally, as part of the repair protocol for an acute injury (such as a broken arm or torn ligament), the body "borrows" stem cells from the bones surrounding the trauma source.

So, if you partially tear one of the tendons in your knee, instead of waiting for the natural blood flow, the body may harvest the stem cells from the surrounding bones to promote quicker healing to the area. Over time, the high-stress regions of the body - think shoulders for boxers and knees for runners - become perpetually low on resources as the body is constantly drawing from its stores. MRIs will actually show "hollowed out" sections in athletes and chronic pain patients where previously dense bones have been mined dry.

The good news is when the human body goes into a dramatic period of fasting, our evolutionary programming turns on the stem cell production machines. There is actually a specific gene responsible for sensing an emergency drop in calories. When the gene activates, it turns on an internal survival protocol by producing billions of stem cells in preparation for the lack of nourishment. But in today's world, we rarely take advantage of this natural healing and replenishing process. Instead, we bombard our bodies with daily caloric abundance, leaving our stem cell Lamborghini in the garage unused. I want to be clear that I am speaking of a true fasting period. I do not mean intermittent fasting, or going a day without eating, as described by every wannabe fitness advisor. I mean seventy-two hours or more with very little calories. Not just going to bed and waking up a little hungry. It's when we go into this true survival phase when the body launches the rockets.

This, of course, has caused many people to try to create this magical rebuilding state by intentionally fasting. But what clinical studies and experiments show, however, is that rarely do people in today's world successfully execute a seventy-two hour fast, whether by accident or with intention. Even if we set a rigid goal of fasting for a day or two, we usually cave in. Given the abundance of food and almost unlimited access to calories, few people have the stone-cold will power to make it without breaking open the Doritos bag. This spawned more research and more clinical studies that led to a groundbreaking find. Studies now show that by restricting calories *significantly* and extending the period of time to five days, we can produce the same boost in metabolic repair and stem-cell production. This was the birth of the "Five-Day Fast Mimicking Diet."

I was first introduced to the Fast Mimicking Diet by my doctors at Rocky Mountain Regenerative Medicine in Boulder. I was diagnosed with advanced Osteoarthritis in my pelvis, and the doctors determined that stem cell therapy was the best course of action. But before they harvested my stem cells for processing and reintegration into my pelvis, they put me on the Fast Mimicking Diet to increase my stem cell count. They explained to me that literally billions of cells would be created during the five days.

They were right, and after the treatment, I experienced a huge boost in healing and was able to ride my fat bike a thousand miles from Detroit to New York through the winter, even only just a few weeks after my treatment. The entire experience had so many unexpected benefits that it is still something I do two to three times a year. I immediately started having my own coaching clients implementing the same protocol. It has proven to be an incredibly effective way of not just healing our sputtering metabolisms, but also in creating a connection to how we eat and how our eating habits affect our bodies in a medical setting.

So, just like all my personal coaching clients have done, for the next five days, you are going to be restricting your calories significantly enough to give you all the benefits that your evolutionary biology is capable of. That means eating no more than eight-hundred calories per day for the guys, and for you goddesses a scant six-hundred calories per day. I have done this myself a few times, and I can tell you, if you commit to this fully, it is not as difficult as you might think, but only if you go all in! This five-day period will have benefits that extend way past the microbiological symphony being conducted on the cellular level inside your bones. You are going to learn about how little you need to eat compared to how much you *think* you need to eat. You will find that if you start to economize calories, you can really stretch your meals.

The last time I did the Five-day Fast Mimicking Diet, I purchased three medium-sized containers of spinach and a tub of hummus for *each day*. If you divide a hummus container into thirds and combine each portion into one of the spinach containers and then close the lid and vigorously shake it to mix the hummus in, you get three quite large-sized meals for the day, still leaving you fifty to one-hundred calories left for an apple or banana as a snack. Get creative, read labels, and poke around a little, and you'll see that if you strip things down to the basics, you can get through this reasonably comfortably. After the first couple of days, it starts to feel totally normal. So that brings us to the heart of step three - create a five-day meal plan and start your ritual healing.

During this five-day healing, we are going to place more emphasis on meditation. Make it a priority to meditate twice a day during this time, once in the morning and again at night. I will give you five separate meditation focuses, and I caution you to treat this period as a very spiritual time. Resist the temptation to look at this as a weight-loss period if you can. Instead, place importance on the healing aspect of it. Remind yourself that it is okay to be hungry. Try to detach yourself from the emotional part of hunger and be willing to sit and take inventory on how you feel before you take any action.

Day one meditation: Find a reason that's bigger than any doubt or temptation for you to break your commitment to this program.

Day two meditation: Look deep inside yourself for a deep well of undiscovered strength.

Day three meditation: Reaffirm the reasons for this rehab. Remind yourself of what led you to start this journey.

Day four meditation: Celebrate how far you have come!

Day five meditation: Remember what you have learned. Find your takeaway lessons from this five-day healing ritual that you can use moving forward.

A note for any athletes that are currently training for an event… suck it up and stay on the path. Keep training. The more you train, the better the effect will be for you. But I will warn you - I was training three hours a day for bike races the last time I did the five-day fast, and on day four, my training fell apart. But if you stick to it, and just let your workouts suffer for a couple of days, or even stop training if you need to, you'll be fine. Do not go over your calorie allotment, that's non-negotiable. If you go over the calorie allotment, the gene that monitors starvation will turn off, the stem cell boost will end abruptly, and you will have negated the effects.

Intention 5

The Fast Mimicking Diet is over. You made it. You're probably feeling lighter, stronger, and very in-tune to what you eat. If you didn't do the five-day challenge, go back and do it. If you did navigate the bumpy terrain, and you're like me, you might even be afraid to start eating more. If so, it's natural to want to keep the momentum going once you feel the pounds coming off. I want you to keep that fire burning and fueling you for the rest of your journey, but I also want to caution you not to make this period of time too extreme. If you go too crazy, you'll run the risk of crashing and burning in an epic fail. Either way, whether you are one-hundred percent ready to eat more or if you are feeling tentative about adding back additional calories, it should be obvious to you that you cannot live long-term on six-hundred or eight-hundred calories per day.

Since this book is primarily focused on combating your food addiction and less focused as being a specific weight-loss book, I am going to leave it to you on how you want to proceed in terms of calorie intake. I think for most people, something in the fifteen-hundred to the two-thousand range for weight-loss is healthy. If you are focused *only* on restoring your eating to a healthy and sustainable practice, do not overly concern yourself with calories from now on. Simply focus on the quality of the food you are eating and remain solid in the parameters of the WFPB universe. Keeping in mind the last five days should have driven home the point that you need *way* less food than you think you do, and if you ultimately want to bring your weight number down, you will need to create a caloric deficit.

In the interest of keeping you from launching into a murderous rage in the near future, I want to remind you it took a long time to put on that stored fat, and it will take a little effort and time to take it off too, so relax and try to be patient. Furthermore, I want to bring your attention to the reality that the effort to remove the stored fat on your body is an entirely different undertaking than the long-term maintenance of a new and healthy body. Many times, without realizing it when we start a weight-loss program, we immediately try to jump right to a lifestyle that includes an abundance of healthy food. This is a great plan for once we get to our weight goal, but to get there, we have to create a deficit. We cannot skip over the work that needs to be done and arrive immediately at a new norm. We must generate an increased internal demand that will result in the body removing stored fat.

Rest assured that during this rehab we are integrating behaviors, thoughts, and practices that will allow you to live all your remaining days without the constant battle with food, *but* if you want to achieve massive weight-loss (fifty or one-hundred pounds or more), you will to need to double down on the physical intensity that is coming later in this program to get that lean and natural state that you desire.

The caloric deficit required for weight-loss is not predicated on one area alone and is accomplished in a multitude of ways. As I have hopefully laid out for you, this program is designed to re-wire your body so that it will be more naturally predisposed to burn more calories and sustain itself on fat. But while that is happening, you must eat clean, and endeavor to eat slightly less than you think you need. We must move and train our bodies through physical work. I am going to resist speaking to the physical odyssey that you will be embarking on until later in the program, so for now, just remember to eat WFPB items only. Eat fewer calories than you think you need, and give yourself fully the ritual of this rehab. Do the meditations, become present in your journaling, and do not give free rent in your head to the demons that may pop up to tell you that you can't do this.

Your homework for today is to watch the documentary movie *Game Changers*. Afterward, take some time to reflect, deliberately and mindfully, what you will be eating for the remaining days of the program. You don't have to map out every meal perfectly - although that's a solid plan for success - but you should have a firm idea of how many calories and what types of meals you will be constructing. If you are at a loss, I'll nudge you again to invest a couple of minutes on Google checking out "simple WFPB meals," poke around the "Forks Over Knives" Facebook group (you'll find me there as well) and devote some extra effort to finding some menus and recipes that fit into your brain. Being comfortable and confident is a huge insurance plan against those speed bumps that threaten to slow you down.

Do not let this day come to an end without writing in your journal. Try to sketch out how you feel as you come off your calorie restriction. Devote ten minutes to working on your breathing. Do not negotiate with the voices in your head that tell you this is insignificant. The meditations have gravity for your rehabilitation - the "pull everything together." After all, those voices are the ones that made you so sick to begin with. Those nagging suggestions brought destruction and depression hidden in the coat pockets of their comfortable embrace.

Intention 6

Previously, I gave you some wiggle room on your diet choices. Now I am going to reel you back in just a little with an "extra credit" project. While I do think you are safe moving forward, as long as you remain vigilant and committed to constructing your meals with WFPB bricks, I also want you to have some sort of scaffolding to stand on instead of hanging off the building by one hand while trying to build your new life with the other. So… if you care to dig deeper - let's create a menu.

Your menu should include three breakfast selections, three lunch choices, and three dinner ideas.

I am not going to do this for you, but I will help. The act of researching, deliberating, and ultimately writing out the menu is as important as the finished product. Remember, you must remain willing to do the things you wouldn't previously do if you want results you've never had.

Breakfast presents for many people the biggest challenge. Most people are so programmed to eat eggs, bacon, dairy, or other animal products that it feels that the WFPB diet is the wrecker of mornings - it is not. If you aren't quite ready to break free of the tractor full of old farmer-style breakfast images, I suggest you try the tofu and veggie scramble in the next section. But you can also explore chia seed puddings, steel-cut oatmeal, or fruit and protein smoothies as options. Do a little due diligence, and you'll find something that will energize and excite you. Add three different breakfast ideas to your menu.

Lunch is often the trickiest meal of the day. For many of us, our time usually isn't our own, work schedules are nuts, and if you don't plan it out, you might end up at a restaurant of your co-worker's choice, or skipping lunch, or any number of potential food disasters. I can't speak to what your particular mid-day obstacles are, but I am one-hundred percent sure you can overcome them easily if you put your head to it. There is no such thing as a work environment that is conducive only to destructive food choices.

When I was losing weight in 2005, just two weeks into my journey, I started a new job that consisted of hanging out in state fairs, home shows, airports, and hotels for weeks at a time with a constant flux of change and unpredictability. My solution was to prepare whole wheat tortillas with peanut butter and banana, cut them in half, and put them into Ziploc bags. I prepared these in my hotel room and carried them in my backpack. I became quite accustomed to this practice after a while and even found myself eating the same way at home. Eventually, I branched out with my dietary choices, but there was comfort in the predictability and repetition of eating this way every day.

My point is we can always find a way, and this was my way. Your way will be totally different, but I am sure you can come up with a solid plan. Oh, and I want to throw out there that grocery stores are lunch options… you do not have to go to restaurants. You can always hit up the supermarket on a whim. Even if you find yourself held hostage by fast-food terrorists that will shoot your ass dead for noncompliance, you can always get a Veggie Delight at Subway, or a rice and beans salad bowl at Chipotle. Write down three lunch options that fit into your world.

Dinner. Ah yes, the most glorious and least important meal of the day. As you know, by now, I like to stir up lots of things, including the shit from time to time. The reason I call dinner the least important meal is because, by the time the dinner rolls are passed around for most people, the day is over. I'm not sure when our meal planning diverged from the practical to the social cortices of our minds, but at some point, we stopped eating based on how we live and started eating based on how we interact.

In the earliest days of our country, we ate based on the structure of our days. Most people were farmers or tradesmen that rose early in the day and worked hard until sunset. As a result, we would rise, eat our largest meal of the day - breakfast. The sustenance was needed to provide energy for the day's chores. We broke in the afternoon for the second largest meal of the day - lunch. Finally, after the work was done, we ate a sensible dinner - not too much or we wouldn't sleep well - and then we repeated the process the next day. We ate based on what we were *going* to do, not in response to what we *did*.

As our cities grew and our careers and family structures started to evolve, our eating patterns adapted in response. We began to separate from the antiquated model that featured houses and farms being a central part of our lives, as we scattered from the farm to the universities and the metro areas. Then we started using our minds to provide for our families as we used to rely on our muscles. As a result of this separation from the traditional routine, the dinner table became more of a daily reunion. It became the only place where mom, dad, and the kids saw each other during the day. The dinner table became as much about keeping the family together socially as it was a time to eat. The unplanned aftermath of this practice is the traditional American dinner. What used

David Clark

to be a small last meal of the day has become more of a Thanksgiving-like feast. Large plates of multiple dishes, meats, breads, veggies, and of course, dessert. Every night. No wonder we are so fat.

Today even professional athletes fall prey to a practice of eating large meals after a hard training effort to "recover" from the damage of training. Yet we know that the human body is only able to biologically appropriate a small portion of calories (two-hundred-fifty to five-hundred) directly to our muscles from a post-workout meal. So, the notion that we need a proportionately large meal after a hard effort is false. This was an idea that was born of marketing sleight of hand, not nutritional science. Eating a large meal at the end of the day when our metabolic and biological function is slowing down, makes it more likely that the body will get excess calories.

We are going to correct this error by reframing our meals, by choosing to see our eating patterns in a new way, and by thinking of eating as fueling for the activity that is to come. In other words, I need you to start to eat for what you will be doing over the next three to four hours, not the previous three to four hours. This should result in your dinners becoming substantially less than previously consumed. You will find this practice fits perfectly into the design and application for the machine that is you. Your biological and metabolic functions will start to pick up momentum. Your hunger, hormonal levels, blood chemistry, and cognitive function will all improve, and you will just fucking feel better.

After you design your menu, hit that cushion and work on your breathing for ten minutes. Just you and your breathing. Deep inhale, slow exhale...

MEDITATION

You are what you eat - literally. Every cell in your body is made from all the nutrients that comprise your diet. Everything you put in your body is important, and food is not your pleasure delivery mechanism. You eat to fuel the miracle machine that is you. You wouldn't dream of absentmindedly poisoning the temple that holds your essence. The program is not about diets or weight-loss. It's about healing, and it's about becoming whole.

ACTION

Walk, run, or cycle. Move your body with intention for at least thirty minutes three to four times per week. Break a sweat, no leisurely strolls at the mall.

NUTRITIONAL INSPIRATION (Five-Day Ritual)

Breakfast - Two pieces of low-calorie toast with low-calorie sugar-free fruit spread
Lunch - Container of spinach with your choice of hummus
Dinner - Container of kale with beans and salsa.

Before going on to the next stage of rehab, you should have:

- *Cleaned out your kitchen*
- *Gone shopping for nutritious WFPB foods*
- *Completed the 5-day Fast Mimicking Diet*
- *Started a journal*
- *Started to meditate*
- *Investigated and researched WFPB recipes*
- *Created a menu*
- *Watched **Game Changers** Documentary*

STAGE 2

Chapter 8
Unfuck Your Mind

"The more you know yourself, the more you forgive yourself."
- Confucius

STEP FOUR

"I faced all my demons with pen and paper in hand."

Let's be honest. Before you started this program, you were kind of fucked. Death was chasing you from your dinner plate. There might have only been a fleeting understating of this, something you brushed up against late at night while lying in bed, but you felt it. Like looking into the corner of the dark room and seeing a shadowy figure hiding there. But instead of investigating, you simply rolled over and shut your eyes, hoping that it was just a trick of the light. But like in *Gerald's Game* by Stephen King, one day, you came to realize that there actually *was* a monster lurking in the corner staring at you and that there was something deeply wrong in the house of you.

What you thought you knew about food was fucking you, what people have told you about why you overeat was fucking you, and, more importantly, how you saw yourself and how you saw the world was fucking you. But by successfully completing the first stage of this program, you stopped the fucking. That means you are no longer at this moment getting hammered on. But… now we need to undo the damage that your thoughts, beliefs, and practices have caused. Unlike real life, in *this* journey, you can unfuck yourself all the way back to virginity.

Now that I have reached my obscenity allotment for the remainder of the book, let's put to rest for a while the topic of *how* you ended up here. Maybe you do have a genetic predisposition to addiction. There might even be a gene that causes you to get caught in the cycle of self-medicating with food. But even if that's true, even if addiction is a real disease, that is not going to help you get better. What we need to explore is what causes you to *stay* here… What are you hiding from when you look to food for comfort? What is going on inside you that causes you to eat in a way that is out of sync with your biological and evolutionary psychology?

Do you remember how liberating it was to pull all that garbage out of your refrigerator? How oddly peaceful it was to see the wholesome food inside the new sparkling clean appliance? Well, that's exactly what we are going to do with your head. We are going to pull out all the garbage that has been rotting behind the empty Tupperware containers in your mind. We are clearing out all the junk food and leaking condiment bottles of your emotional pain, placing it on the floor in the light of day, and then throwing it all away.

I know that might seem really scary. Trust me - I know. But this is where this program is really going to take a sharp turn from the practical to the radical. By definition, that means to help to really hit the spiritual root of the problem. I am going to push you to see your pain. To hold your pain like a child and then release your pain and allow it to become something new. I am going to lead you down a winding road that will ultimately expose how you currently view yourself, help you see what is holding you back, and finally help you change into the person you've always wanted to be. But to get there, you have to DO THE WORK.

This is where this book becomes a real-life treatment program and not just a behavioral change story. Make no mistake; it is also the process that will ultimately save you from your destructive relationship with food, which navigates much of the same path that every addict must undergo to achieve recovery. I am not just talking about abstaining from overeating. I am talking about creating a peaceful way of living that is so amazing that you'd never dream of walking away from it. A place where you don't feel the need to seek comfort from food, and where you would never poison yourself willingly with junk food.

Before you put up the "I am not an alcoholic or true addict" defense, let me state that although the spiritual work we are getting ready to do is paramount to saving the addict, it's also something that *every* single human being on the planet should do. That is if they want to become truly happy. Addicts do not have the market cornered on being lost, frustrated, and unfulfilled. We all suffer silently, and this program can heal the broken heart that is hiding behind every shallow smile you see in the world.

Start by writing down everything you can think of that has been holding you down. Write down the worst things that you have done. Write down the worst and most shameful moments of your life. Write down the times when you felt the least human. Write down the things you fear facing. Write down the things that you have made a life practice to hide from. I know this is painful, and as humans, we have spent a great portion of our lives trying to bury and ignore precisely these memories. But you must drag these demons into the light of day now.

You have been carrying the pain far too long, and it isn't serving you. We all have these experiences; we all have ghosts in the attic. No matter how deeply you think you have buried them, trust me, they still haunt you. Not following through on my own inventory, the first time I tried, it cost me over ten years of my life. When I first went to Alcoholics Anonymous and was told I needed to face down my demons, I walked out shaking my head. "No way - fuck that." So, instead of getting better, I got worse. I kept carrying that pain. I kept telling myself that the things that happened in my life had no hold over me.

"That shit is in the past; I don't think about it at all! How can it be hurting me?" I lamented. "If I relive all that shit, it *will* hurt!" That is the point. If we ever hope to be free, we must dig up the bodies in the backyard.

When I finally went to work on my inventory, I started with some of the light grievances of my past. We all have things that aren't buried too deep and yet cause us pain in times of reflection. Some harsh words I said to my mom. The times I lied and shoplifted as a kid. I started to write down how my selfish tendencies have caused pain to my ex-wife. How my eating was affecting my loved ones. How my health was limiting my time and what habits my kids were learning from seeing how I live.

Then I started to dig deeper. I remembered how I ruined Christmas one year by getting so drunk I couldn't wrap gifts for my family. I remembered how I placed my own destructive habits over everyone else. It took a long time, but I eventually started to think of what I call "the darkroom." The room in my mind that I had locked up so tightly. The door that I had been shoving furniture up against in a desperate effort make sure light was never cast past the threshold of its entrance. The room of my childhood. The room that held my deepest pain. The pain that came from never feeling safe. The pain that came from despite having two of the most amazing loving parents in the world, I never felt like I was a viable member of the world. The pain of how I felt bullied, how I felt left behind, and how I felt abused...

David Clark

because, I *was* abused. I *had* been hurt. By the worst possible offender. Someone I trusted.

For my whole life, I had been hiding from the fact that I was sexually abused starting at just five years old. Not just a single occurrence of abuse, but a long practice that lasted for years. For all my adult years, I keep telling myself it wasn't real. That I chose it. That I welcomed it somehow. Here is the part that was so important to me, and that is important to *you* now... what happened to me was not the reason for all my pain. It was not the reason that I sought comfort from food, drugs, and alcohol. It was the fact that I buried it - *that* was the real demon. That's what fueled my destruction.

Demons feed on darkness and silence. The more we bury them, and the more we act as if they aren't real, the stronger they get. Those bastards all breathe the same poison regardless of what spawned them. I have seen simple resentment cause people to lose years of their lives as the weight of small transgression grows stronger and stronger in their mind. I have seen a lack of affection, verbal abuse, and being abandoned in a grocery store cause as much damage as physical or sexual abuse. So, don't judge or score your own experiences. Do NOT minimize what you've been through. Just make sure you shine light into every corner of your heart.

It's okay if you cannot make the connection between your emotional pain and your dinner plate. You are going to feel a huge weight come off your shoulders by doing this regardless of the future effects. When I was done with the process, I felt as if I had never experienced a free day in my life. As if I spent my whole life in prison until one day, the warden came in and unlocked my cage. I walked into a world that I didn't even know existed. Like I handed the universe all my worst fears, my deepest pain, and my most embarrassing moments because I didn't need them anymore. It was the most liberating thing I have ever done, and it makes me cry when I think of all the pain I was carrying for no reason.

Don't worry. I am not one of those people that believes in being a victim. I am not trying to turn you into some kind of brainwashed pussy that will be in therapy for the rest of your life talking about micro-aggressions and safe spaces. I am talking about doing the warrior's work here. Identifying your enemy. Challenging your demons to a fucking fistfight in the middle of town. Going to battle for a new life. Not being willing to "eek" through life getting the shit kicked out of you until you die. That's what we are doing here.

So now it's your time. Time for you to climb out of your grave. So, grab the biggest shovel you can find and dig deeply. There is no right or wrong way to do this. You are simply looking to expose all the things that keep you up at night. The things you feel you could never share. The things that you would be mortified if people knew… be fearless. Be thorough and stay mindful that this will ultimately be giving you a feeling of freedom that every human deserves to have, but few ever will.

David Clark

Intention 7

The inventory you are doing continues. There is no way to be able to successfully purge the weight of your past in a twenty-four-hour period. So even if you feel you have scrubbed down the floor, go back and look for more dirt. Think forensics. You washed away the mud and dust, now go get the fingerprints and DNA. Try to expand the window into your past. Explore your deepest fears. What are you most afraid of? What is the worst thing you fear happening to you?

Take a walk and let these thoughts take root. Try to be alone in your mind. If you are like most people, you aren't very good at doing nothing. By the end of this program, I hope to have helped you eliminate the conflict that starts to surface when you stop moving. This inventory is the first step in releasing the pressure of the spiritual steam that's been building in the boiler room of you.

When you do your ten minutes of breathing today, instead of directing your thoughts to your breath, I want you to focus on your inventory work. Let the thoughts you've been hiding from sit in front of you. Don't judge them or argue with them. Just let them exist. I only want you to be present with them. Observe your thoughts as they take form from afar as if they are not even yours. Treat them like they are a random person's deepest moments that you merely are observing. They aren't bad or good. They are simply truth. After the meditation, write in your journal.

Intention 8

Today, we are going to begin the process of building on the foundation you've poured with your breathing exercises. Every inhalation and exhalation served a purpose, and now your goal is to take those powerful emissions and form them into a solid meditation practice. Today, you are going to start using meditation to help connect to the center of your being. In Buddhism, they call it "Buddha Nature," which speaks to the energy that lies at the center of who you are. We all have the potential to be Buddhas, to be enlightened, and awaken our lives. So, get on your cushion and let me guide you.

I want you to read this paragraph with a meditative mind. I want you to imagine how you will be meditating as you read this. Set your timer for fifteen minutes. Sit upright. Straighten your back and relax your hands and feet. Start to focus on your breathing. Take many deep breaths, as you have in your previous sessions. When you feel relaxed and reasonably focused, I want you to start allowing yourself to feel the weight of your past leaving you with every exhale. Focus only on your breath as you deeply inhale, then allow your body to fall into a deep and peaceful state as you feel the dark energy of your pain leaving you. Feel the way your body relaxes and resets as you exhale all the things you've been holding onto. You don't need your pain anymore. Think of this as an almost surgical session. It isn't just a spiritual ritual; you are actually cutting the painful memories from your mind.

Make no mistake: Your thoughts are as real as the floor beneath you. All that happens in the vivid richness of your mind is a projection from within. There is nothing solid around you, just photons, quarks, atoms, and particles whizzing around you at the speed of light. Your mind is interpreting those things as "chair, floor, house." But they are only real because of the chemicals in your mind. So, when you release the part of your mind holding on to pain, in a very real way, the pain itself is gone.

Continue to allow yourself to go deeper and deeper into the previously unnoticed hiding places inside you. Turn on an imaginary light inside you and sweep the house for any clutter. When your time is done, create a precise picture in your mind's eye of you shutting the lights down in a completely secure, safe, and clean house. This house is your mind. It is clear. You can rest well now. The monsters are gone.

You are now free of the conflict that was tormenting you. Wasn't it really the conflict about your identity that was haunting you even more than the memories themselves? If you have lived these terrible things, does that mean you a terrible person? Are you unworthy of love? Will people discover who you truly are and judge you?

If being in a thousand group therapy rooms over the years has taught me anything, it's that we all have the same fears. We might not have the same exact stories, but the internal narrative of those stories is all in the same voice. I have seen hundreds of people at their wit's end, on the brink of a total breakdown, in desperate exasperation, finally expose their deepest fears to a group of strangers. You can see the shame in their eyes, the total vulnerability as they expect to be judged for all the horrible things they have been holding onto.

Instead, they look up and see knowing and welcoming eyes. They see people that understand what they've been holding onto. Sexual abuse, trauma, cheating, and violence have almost the exact effect on the soul as lying, being selfish, and having narcissistic traits. It's not the things we do that hurt us; it's the fear of being less than everyone else. But we are all on the same path here. We have all been hurt. We are all trying our best. The fact that you are here now shows that you are ready to heal - and that is what's happening to you now. That's what the tears mean.

MEDITATION

You are the cause of all the pain in your life, and it is you that needs to change. More specifically, your thoughts and how you choose to see things need to change. Where you are is not bad luck, it is not your childhood, nor is it the result of what has happened in your life. You are not your past. You are not the things that have happened to you. Your body is not you. Your mind is not you. The true you is only energy. That

David Clark

energy has never been hurt. It's never done wrong. The true energy of you is unscathed and ready for you to heal and to let go of your pain.

ACTION

Walk, run, or cycle. Move your body with intention for at least forty-five minutes three to four times a week. Break a sweat, no leisurely strolls at the mall.

NUTRITIONAL INSPIRATION

Tofu Scramble - Start with silken or soft tofu. Lightly (and I mean lightly) spray the cooking pan with some coconut cooking spray, squish the tofu into the pan with a large spoon, add veggies of your choice (mushrooms, green peppers, onions, etc.). Mix every 2-3 minutes for 12 minutes and serve. As with all cooking efforts, you will need to experiment with spices (salt, pepper, Mrs. Dash, etc.) to avoid a bland morning meal.

STEP FIVE

"I spoke my truth to the universe."

Guess what? You are human. Which means that you possess every characteristic of the very best of our species. From Martin Luther King, Jr. to Mother Teresa - their same spirit of love lives in all of our DNA. It also means that as humans, we possess the worst of human traits as well. We all lie. We all cheat. We all hurt other people, and we have all been hurt, too. The thing that determines the ultimate quality of who we are is how much we are willing to grow and not how low we have fallen. To be able to move on from the last step, you must truly accept this truth. The purpose of the inventory was to allow you to clean out the refrigerator of your mind. To take out the garbage, as it were.

In our lives, all that we do and all that happened to us has had a lasting effect on how we interact in the world. They are not permanent effects, but they do not go away on their own, either. Has a song or a movie caused you to relive a painful memory instantly? Has the mere sight of a familiar street corner or the smell of a particular cologne instantly touched your emotions and altered your mental state? This is called a "Samskara."

"Samskaras are psychological imprints on our spirit, and they are a basis for the development of the karma theory. In Buddhism, the Sanskrit term Samskara is used to describe "formations."

David Clark

According to various schools of Indian philosophy, every action, intent, or preparation by an individual, leaves a Samskara in the deeper structure of a person's mind. These impressions then await volitional fruition in that individual's future, in the form of hidden expectations, circumstances, or a subconscious sense of self-worth.
These Samskaras manifest as tendencies, karmic impulses, subliminal impressions, habitual potencies, or innate dispositions. In ancient Indian texts, the theory of Samskara explains how and why human beings remember things and the effect that memories have on people's suffering, happiness, and contentment." (Wikipedia)

By definition, everything you wrote down in your inventory is Samskara. You simply would not have remembered it or thought to write it down if it didn't leave a deep impression in your mind to begin with. Like a vampire, these vermin have been feasting off of your spiritual blood for years. But just like a vampire, these past karmic scars cannot survive the light of day. By dragging them into the sun's warmth, you have erased the hypnotic trance they've held over you. I'm not saying you won't have to remind yourself of your emancipation - you will. But unless you choose to rewrite them into your mind by reliving them over and over, they are dead. So, let's release the pain from your orbit and let them float away into space.

I want you to take those inventory pages you created in step four, all the pain you could press from

the seeds of your past and read them out loud –
literally, audibly and loudly. I want you to read
exactly what you wrote down. Read them literally as
you have them written and then read it again, adding
and changing to expand on the thoughts. Do not read
them tentatively, read them with confidence and
purpose. Let's face it, you're half-crazy already, so
having a conversation with yourself won't really take
you someplace you haven't already been. The act of
reading out loud is significant. You must take these
memories from the loosely tangible thoughts
represented on the pages and release them out of your
mind through your voice. Bear witness to all that you
have endured. You have identified the wounds, and
now is the time to rip the Band-Aids off so the scabs
can fully heal.

You are not just releasing the Samskaras from
their resting place in your soul. You are forgiving
yourself for all your own past transgressions. You are
releasing the pain and all the dominoes that have
fallen as a result of your pain - the pain that landed on
others. You have been hurt, and as a result, it's caused
you to hurt others. This is what it means to be human.
All humans deserve to be free to reinvent themselves
and to create a new karma singularity, that will bring
a "Big Bang" into a new life.

A quick note on karma - it doesn't work in the
way that most people think of it. It is not a tally sheet
or a running debt that you are accruing. The universe
isn't going to punish you or reward you based on your
actions. This is a very Western or secular notion of

David Clark

how the universe works. It might make sense if instead of spiritual beings, you and I were some sort of universal accountants, but I am quite sure that if you kick a baby and then immediately hug an orphan, you aren't "back to zero."

I believe karma to be something we are changing and creating in every moment, which is not ironically what the experience of life itself is. At the risk of drifting too far out into the ocean of spiritual thought, time itself is a human construct. Horses in the field do not compare today's rainy weather to yesterday's sunshine. The seasons do not subscribe to daylight savings, and the oceans really are not concerned with the clock. No, it is not time, but the moon and gravity that dictate how the tides behave. The only reason we parse our experience into days and years is because humans decided to arbitrarily count how many times the planet revolves around the sun. But under these rules, time itself would be entirely different on other planets. When you consider that a day on Saturn is just over ten hours long, you see that the whole idea of time is completely irrelevant to the experience of life.

The reality is that nothing exists outside of the present moment. The sun has no memory of yesterday, and the stars have no hope for tomorrow. When you get down to the quantum reality of human life, you and I are only lucid in the miracle of now. Although it seems we can most certainly get lost in yesterday's fond reflection or the warm promise of tomorrow, we are only touching that with today's mind, and only from the present moment's perspective.

What we think of as the past is really only the memory of a memory, a recollection of a story we have told ourselves over and over again. We have no solid connection to what happens behind us. We were all once babies. At one time, we all stood three feet tall. But can you really recollect your toddler experience? Can you even see yesterday in a meaningful way? We can't even create in any tangible way the exact moments of earlier today, much less years ago. Tomorrow is a never-ending, never fulfilled promise. No one has ever lived a tomorrow. Everything you have ever experienced and everything you *will* experience will happen through the prism of "right now."

So, relax, and take comfort in the fact that karma isn't the ledger entry of our balance sheet. You aren't carrying the past. Instead, like life, karma is something we are creating in front of us. As we step on the brick of today, tomorrow's brick vanishes. Along this sidewalk of reality, there are no bricks in front of us; they only materialize as our feet hit the ground. The things we do affect only the very next thing. If we keep doing the same things, we are stuck. If we do something new, a new life instantly starts to form. The karma we are currently creating can last forever, becoming darker and darker, or it can become as bright as the sun in a single thought. We choose what happens to us by choosing what we do now. Do

David Clark

not let the lies of yesterday tell you anything different.

Intention 9

Consider this intention a check-in, or even better a check*up*. Go back and read your journal in its entirety. Also, re-read the previous steps of this rehab program if you can. Go back and make sure that you have given yourself to all the tasks. Make sure you aren't asleep at the wheel of your rehab. Negotiating the terms with yourself for complete capitulation is part of the process.

If you are like most people, you have likely become accustomed to going through the motions. You glance at something quickly and pull out what you deem to be the important parts. But that's not how growth works. The greatest athletes are the ones that are coachable. The talented prodigy rarely lasts long in sports because they have failed to develop the desire to be humble and continue to improve. My long-standing definition of humility is precisely *the willingness to take advice against your initial instinct to dismiss it.* That is where all the wisdom is hiding.

It's probably felt a bit like an emotional roller coaster over the last several days. It's probably felt like a lot more downs than ups. For your meditation today, set the timer for fifteen minutes. If, for some reason, you have skipped over the mediation part of the program, go back and do them now!

Open with a few minutes on your breathing. Settle your mind and bring your focus to it. As you start to feel more peaceful, I want you to start searching for strength. Reach out with your emotions and your mind and seek positive energy. Try to feel powerful, indestructible. I want you to breathe deeply and feel yourself becoming an inseparable part of all the energy around you. The ocean, the wind, the stars are all living in you.

Intention 10

When was the last time you went for a long walk? When I was at the pinnacle of my ultra-running career, I would run one-hundred to one-hundred-twenty miles every week. Using my body as a means for travel was a regular part of my life. I ran to business meetings, my kid's hockey games, and even to the gym to workout. Yet, I rarely just went for a walk. Once, while I was on a trip to New York, I left my hotel and just walked around the city. I couldn't believe how deeply introspective the experience was.

I have written an entire book on the spirituality of running. It's a topic I have explored intimately. Yet I feel walking is its own means of spiritual travel. It has its own unique way of communicating with the soul and the environment. It's an internal ocean to be discovered, providing a vast and diverse ecosystem for processing our thoughts and feelings. The Tibetans believed that to achieve redemption, embarking on a long trek on foot was necessary. This meant days and weeks of walking to achieve the needed reconciliation for spiritual rebirth. They believed the greater the redemption that was desired, the longer the walk must be.

Today, you are going to set aside some time for a long walk. At least an hour and preferably more if you can. There is no agenda for your pilgrimage. The only parameter is that you don't extensively plan it. If you choose to go to a park or mountain - great. But don't draw out a course or choose the exact route. Just treat it like a meditation of sorts. Let it unfold as it wants to. Be present in the steps. Let your mind relax. Connect to your breathing and just let your mind press the journey. If you didn't realize it yet, you are on one hell of a life-changing voyage, might as well let your legs stretch out as your mind does the same.

MEDITATION

Be patient. Much of your internal storm rages because your mind is never still. Learn to let go of the need to control everything around you. You are not the general manager of the universe. You do not need to argue every point. You do not need to overthink everything. You do not need to be right. Become willing to be an observer in your life and the lives of others. Let things happen in their own time. Resist your usual reaction to do and say things in the moment. Allow some space for your thoughts and actions to form before you pull the trigger.

ACTION

Walk, run, or cycle. Move your body with intention for at least forty-five minutes three to four times a week. Break a sweat, no leisurely strolls at the mall.

NUTRITIONAL INSPIRATION

WeAreSuperman's Power Pasta - Start with pasta of your choice. I like spinach pasta, or any pasta made from veggies (you can find this at almost any grocery store) and cook pasta as directed. Put pasta in a baking dish and add pasta sauce. Add finely chopped broccoli, diced garlic, and cubed avocado. Sprinkle some nutritional yeast (found at any health food store) over the top and bake at 375 degrees for 45 minutes.

David Clark

STEP SIX

"I burned the bridge to my past and forgave myself for being human."

Step six is divided into two parts - A and B.

PART A

I'm sure if you look back to your fearless inventory, you probably didn't feel much like an accountant when you made it. It likely didn't feel as if you were simply counting and writing down your thoughts. You probably felt more like a prosecutor. Like you were digging up evidence, deposing the witnesses of your past, and presenting opening arguments in the potential conviction of the State of Humanity vs. You. That is certainly how I felt when I saw my own bloody fingerprints in the crime scene of my past. So, if the inventory process made you feel like a defendant, now it's time for the defense to present its case.

Therefore, I need you to reframe all the things from your inventory in a way that mitigates or explains your actions. Walk the jury through the circumstances surrounding the acts in question. Show the human side of the defendant (you). I know in my own court proceeding, I had to explain to the jury that all my crimes were committed in the presence of terrible childhood experiences and that even though I had two loving parents, I was abused by a trusted friend.

I grew up feeling like the world was the place where everyone else lived, and I wasn't welcome to join them. I had to explain that underneath all the ego, the controlling, selfish, manipulating behavior that I inflicted on even those closest to me, I was just a frightened little boy. I was afraid that everyone was better than me, and when I lashed out, it was just me I was fighting - not them.

I was lost in a world where I couldn't stop eating and drinking myself to death, even though eating and drinking made me feel even worse. I was broken. When I saw myself as just a hurt human being, it made it quite easy to finally forgive myself. Now it's your turn. Mount a great defense. Your future is depending on it. For this case, you need to be Perry-fucking-Mason.

Once you have made your case, write it down and submit the document to your journal. If you were honest and open, the evidence should be overwhelming in your favor. You aren't a violent offender in the jurisprudence of humanity. You were simply a person trying to navigate the best you could in a tough situation. If you need to go back and restate your case, do it. If you are battling the notion that you truly are someone beyond reprehension and undeserving of forgiveness, I will submit for you an argument of my own.

David Clark

If you truly were a malignant narcissist with no redeeming qualities at all, you would not be here. You would not be trying to become a better person. There *are* those souls that seem to have no human empathy at all, that seek only to hurt and tear through the world without a single glance backward. Those people would never dream of buying a book like this. To be awake and aware of the possibility that you've done harm is proof of the quality of your heart.

I am reminded of the story of a young monk and an old monk who were walking down the road having a conversation. They were speaking about the pilgrimage they were both currently undertaking - a ritual cleaning of the body and soul. A sacred period of time when monks pledged to bathe five times a day, and they were not allowed to touch or engage in any impure thoughts or actions.

As they were walking down the road, they came across a prostitute who needed some help to cross a shaky bridge. The older monk picked up the woman and carried her across the bridge without a word. He bid her good day on the other side and kept walking. After several miles, the younger monk finally spoke up.

"How could you carry that prostitute during this the purest time of our entire year?"

The older monk replied, "I carried her across the bridge. You have been carrying her ever since then."

It's time to stop carrying the past into today. It's time to move on.

PART B

Time for the final stage two act. This is perhaps my favorite part of **Radical Rehab** as it is a powerful action that will give you the closure you so desperately need after fighting so valiantly on the battlefield of your past. The trenches are clear, and the war has been won. Now it's time to burn the bridge behind you so that you are never tempted to go back to inventory the dead.

You have written down your fearless inventory. You have spoken the words aloud and taken away their power to hide in the dark ambiguity between thoughts and sounds. Now we will transform those acts permanently in a ritualistic act to display that those memories are combustible - I want you to set your past on fire - literally. Yes, tear out the page from your journal, or print it off your computer, and then burn it. Do it in a way that will create a new imprint on your mind. A ritual, a cleansing. Feel the past ignite with the words. Be safe; I don't want any house, or forest fires started in the name of battling food addiction. But put an actual match to the paper.

MEDITATION

No one gets through life without being hurt and without hurting others. We all bleed red, and we all make mistakes. But the pain we hide hurts us a thousand times more than the pain we feel and release. This program is about searching out the wolves that have been chasing you through the forest.

David Clark

You've always been afraid they would catch you and rip you apart. But the wolves are scary only at night when you cannot see them.

ACTION
Walk, run, or cycle. Move your body with intention for at least forty-five minutes three to four times a week. Break a sweat, no leisurely strolls at the mall.

NUTRITIONAL INSPIRATION
Happy Mac & Cashew Cheese - Place 2 cups of cashews in a bowl filled with water. Allow cashews to soak for 2 hours. Drain cashews and place in a blender. Add 2 tablespoons of nutritional yeast (can be purchased at a health food store) and 1/4 cup almond milk, a pinch of garlic salt, and a pinch of onion powder. Blend until nut mixture becomes a consistent paste. Start with elbow macaroni made from lentils (can be purchased at most grocery stores), cook pasta per instructions. Place cooked and drained pasta in oven baking dish spread cashew cheese (paste) over the pasta, and sprinkle gluten-free breadcrumbs on top. Bake at 375 degrees for 45 minutes.

Before going on to the next stage of rehab, you should have:

- *Completed a complete fearless moral inventory*
- *Learned about Samskara and how emotional pain is stored*
- *Read your inventory out loud*
- *Expanded your meditation practice fifteen minutes every day*
- *Written in your journal every day*
- *Engaged in a difficult physical activity every day*
- *Written a compelling case for your own humanity*
- *Burned your fearless moral inventory*

David Clark

STAGE 3

Chapter 9
Unfuck Your Life

"It is never too late to be what you might have been."
— George Eliot

STEP SEVEN

"I created an entirely new identity."

The Phoenix is the mythical bird that can catch fire and rise from its own ashes and become new. Some legends say it dies in a show of flames and combustion, and others say that it merely dies and decomposes before being born again. Either way, *you* are a Phoenix. Those of us that have jumped onto the path of addiction recovery of any kind have willingly caught ourselves on fire in the hopes that a new and stronger bird will fly over the charred remains of the wreckage of our lives. On my tenth year of recovery, I even had a Phoenix tattooed on my neck. That is your step seven task, to get your own tattoo… I'm kidding, of course. But if you even considered it for a moment, I'm impressed by your commitment.

Seriously though, you are standing almost literally in the ashes of your former life. The charcoal of the pages you set on fire might still be warm at the bottom of your fireplace or backyard fire pit. So, let's spread your wings and display them to the astonishment of your friends and family.

You'll remember from *chapter three* that as humans, it is crucial what we think, what we believe, and what we do are all in sync. That means you cannot permanently alter your habits without changing what you believe. The first thing you start believing in is you, or more specifically, who you are capable of becoming. You can be anything you choose, so now is the time to choose something breathtaking. Imagine a new life that will naturally result in eating healthy, training your body to be supremely fit, and accomplishing all your goals.

"Avatar" is not just the title of a movie about blue people from Pandora. In Hinduism, an Avatar is a manifestation of a deity or released soul in bodily form on earth. As a representation of your future self, I want you to create your own Avatar now. Use your journal and be very specific. What kind of athlete would you be if you were starting your life over? What habits do you wish you displayed? What kind of person would you like to be? Is your Avatar happy? If so, why? How does he or she treat people? Write it all down.

Remember who you are is not your past. You are not locked into any rigid identity. You can change everything about yourself. Your traits, your work ethic, your empathy, your intelligence, your education, your career - all pliable. Spend some time in your meditations, exploring what challenges you and what inspires you.

Once you have caught a glimpse of this "new you," I want you to internalize it. Make it real. But be prepared for the push back. You will tell yourself this is silly. You might question the possibility of this actually working too. God forbid you tell someone else. They might have you tested for drugs.

I wish I could tell you that once you make the choice to leave the old life behind, the new one will happen without effort, but you know that would be a lie. It will be hard, but it will be worth it. Yet, as hard as it is to change, it is not the change itself that is causing us so much pain. It is the *resistance* to the change that is so brutal. It's not the work that is hard. It's being caught between full commitment and the effort that is so unbearable.

Imagine if you were lost in the woods. You have no idea where you are or which direction you should go. Do you go north? Do you go south? Should you stay where you are? Should you build a fire? If you are like most people, the fear would be almost paralyzing. The prospect of making the "wrong" choice would keep you from doing anything. Yet, there is no way of ever knowing what lies to the north or the south without moving. Doing nothing is the only assured lousy outcome. But if instead of being paralyzed, you made up your mind to move in a singular direction, with total commitment, without second-guessing yourself, your chances of finding a path would become inevitable. That is the exact place where you find yourself today. It doesn't matter what direction you choose, but choose it. Own it. Start marching through that forest like you were certain a village was around every bend or behind each tree.

You will have your doubts. That is normal, and it's okay. But giving those doubts a place to live in your head, will ultimately derail you. You must develop a mechanism to stop the endless chatter when the voices come up. It can be anything. Looking at a photo, reminding yourself of what you are losing by living your current life, or literally stopping in your tracks, doing some jumping jacks or running around the block. Before you laugh at those last two, try it next time - you'll find those both to be quite effective at putting a stop to the anxiety.

I've heard many runners say before a big race, "Quitting is not an option," and although I think they mean it, that's total bullshit. Quitting is *always* an option, and if you aren't prepared to deal with the desire to quit - you'll fold the fuck up when you do want to throw in the towel. Feeling frustrated or wanting to quit is just a preconditioned response. It's not real. You don't have to do something just because you think about it. It's not a reflection of your character if you struggle with wanting to quit. Everything we do or think is simply a preconditioned response that has been deeply coded into our idea of self. It's all changeable. One strong choice now, followed by another. The next thing you know, you are in a brand-new life.

David Clark

There was a time when each one of us was just a baby. We had no biases or tendencies. Before we thought of ourselves as a name or before we were told we were "American" or "Irish," we simply experienced the world as colors, sounds, and tactile stimuli. We felt or experienced the world instead of judging it or labeling it - that blank slate is the true nature of our identity. Everything about who we are as adults was taught to us by mom and dad, television, society, and every piece of information we have absorbed. It's not really you at all. Don't get me wrong, you are still in there. Somewhere. You are just buried under all those labels, language, and attachments that make it so hard to communicate internally and to be authentic to our true nature.

So, if you want to break the cycle of responding poorly when times get hard, start recognizing that what you feel isn't real at all, but merely a learned behavior. All you need to do to change that behavior is to be mindful of what is happening when you react. And by making a habit of doing this, it will allow you to overwrite a new behavior in its place, essentially.

I can promise you that my current habits and instinctual responses to life in no way resemble the ones that I carried for nearly forty years. I used to shrink and panic at the thought of the unknown. I used to quit on myself all the time. I used to be a reactionary and dishonest person, which is in stark contrast to my current way of sharing my deepest thoughts with strangers and being unable even slightly to bend the truth. For years, I couldn't seem to break free of the cycle no matter how hard I tried.

Yet, I was the one constructing the prisons that I was unable to break out of. Realizing I was in jail was the first step to breaking out of prison. So, give yourself a break if you have periods of doubt and low motivation, but push into them. Look at these moments as an opportunity to prove once and for all that this is real. This is the time that you finally change. If not now, when? That is the thought that carried me over many of these little potential crises. Do not entertain the idea of failing to make this change a reality. Only live in the solutions to whatever conspires to unwind your new reality.

Commitment is not something we experience in fractional quantities. It is something we either have or something we do *not* have. Yet, for some reason, we indulge in the ludicrous idea that we could be ninety-nine percent committed to something. If you are ninety-nine percent committed to your job - you're shopping around. If you are fifty-fifty on the new diet we just started, you are already looking for a way out. Imagine if your spouse informed you that they were ninety-nine percent committed to your marriage. Would that sound encouraging? Pretty good odds, right? Or would you see the missing one percent as a crisis waiting to happen? I'm guessing ninety-nine percent wouldn't be very comforting to you as he or she headed out of town for a work trip.

As humans, we always accomplish, one-hundred percent of the time, what we place at the top of our list. The problem is we don't always consciously choose what lives at the top of said list. Alcoholics have placed getting drunk as the number one priority, and you can bet your ass it will happen. I've seen drunks on crutches plowing through the snow to get to the bar. Of course, a standout in the world of getting the job done is my friend Pete who once got a DUI while driving his car in reverse to the liquor store when his transmission went out. Can you just imagine the police car pulling up to him as their windshields faced each other while driving in the same direction?

Evolution placed "survival" as the default parameter for our intentions. But even something as deeply derived as self-preservation can be manually overwritten. We see it every day with soldiers, police officers, and first responders who willingly sacrifice their own lives to save strangers. Think about that for a moment. Our survival instinct is so strong that we will fight off bears, walk across deserts, or plunge into icy shark-infested waters to swim away from a sinking ship. Yet that base instinct to live can be overridden by the powerful identity shift that occurs when someone chooses a specific career path.

My point is simply that we can choose what is at the top of our list. We can choose what the body and mind will allocate our resources toward. That means if you make this change the single most important thing in your life, an amazing thing will happen - and you will defend it. You will move, bend, and twist anything that stands in your way until it fits into the picture frame. Before you start saying that sounds a trifle selfish, understand that *is* taking care of yourself. Placing your own physical and spiritual health as your top priority will have a ripple effect that spills perfectly onto all aspects of your life. You will be able to care for other people more, you will be able to connect with people more, and you will inspire others to take care of themselves as well.

When you meditate today, let your mind focus on the picture (or Avatar) of who you want to be. You were born as a source of pure energy. You are the universe expressing itself in a human body. As a human being, you have dominion over who you are. Explore the way it would feel to be that person. Allow yourself to picture how you might look. What it would feel like to move that new body around the house or the gym. Before you move on, make sure you have opened up space for that person to exist. You should be able to describe your Avatar to someone else and have them believe the person is real.

Intention 11

We have talked a lot about the transformation that occurs when you meditate and work on your spiritual self, and it's all true. But there are, of course, many physiological reasons for you to be training your body as well. So, let's draw some much-needed attention to the work you have been doing every day by working out. You *have* been working out, haven't you?

Your long-term success depends on how well you rebuild your physical structure. You cannot let your new spirit dwell in the old broken shell. Now that you are putting pure fuel into the tank by eating only WFPB foods, let's put a big engine in the frame, too, by making you more fit than you have ever been. Think of your body as the most fantastical sports car ever made. Not only is it capable of hitting corners like an Indy car and reaching the end of a quarter-mile like a dragster, but your machine will actually get faster and become more fuel-efficient every time it runs out of gas. So, as you complete this seventh step by creating the new Avatar, that will be your new focus, I also want you to make a mental note to start bringing new intensity to the gym with you every day.

Intention 12

Are there things you have done that you regret? When you did your fearless moral inventory, were there some items on the list that you could atone for with a simple call or email? Grab that journal and start making a list of people that you have wronged, people that would likely feel better if you apologized to them. I'm not asking you to make amends for *all* the wrongs you have done (although that process is quite liberating). I'm only suggesting that if you have people that you have treated poorly, it will clear out some more space in that ever-expanding heart of yours if you give them a shout and say, "Hey, I'm sorry I hurt you... I was dealing with some stuff, and I am trying to do better." Everything you have done so far in this program is about letting go of all the things that have hurt you, and creating a life with nothing to hide, having no fear of who you are underneath and setting your karma to a point that brings you bright and happy days.

When you make these calls or emails, do so without any attachment or expectation. You are not doing this for forgiveness or to bring about any result. You are doing this because it's the right thing to do. If these people do not wish to forgive you, they are under no obligation to do so. You are simply making an effort to repair the damage. This act, if done with a pure intention, will help them release their own Samskara.

Intention 13

If you are new to the idea of working out, did you buy new gym clothes? It's certainly not a requirement, but if you did, it's a good sign that you are already at work to keep your momentum going. I think it was Zig Ziglar who said, "Motivation is like bathing, it doesn't last, so you have to do it every day." Putting together a new playlist for your workouts, buying new clothes, or even watching a motivational movie are all easy and great ways to keep you inspired. Keep in mind that you are not working out to go through the motions. Instead, you are a living work of art. Every time you go to the gym or go for a run, you are painting or sculpting. You are chipping away at the marble each day until one day, the art is there.

MEDITATION

Trust this process. Do not rethink, rehash, and constantly judge this experience. Resist the temptation to continually check in and see if you are getting better. Instead, give yourself to the program. Commit to going the whole way before you evaluate your progress. Whether it is this rehab, running a marathon, or operating a business, you will never get anywhere by constantly questioning what you are doing.

ACTION

With new intensity, walk, run, or cycle. Move your body with intention for at least forty-five minutes four to five times a week. Break a sweat, no leisurely strolls at the mall.

NUTRITIONAL INSPIRATION

Homemade Hummus – (1) 15-ounce can of chickpeas (rinsed and drained), 2 cloves garlic (chopped), 2 to 3 tablespoons fresh lemon juice, 1 teaspoon Bragg Liquid Aminos, 3 tablespoons water. Experiment with flavors by adding ingredients such as garlic, red peppers, habanero, etc. Blend all the ingredients into a thick paste, using a small amount of water as necessary to achieve desired consistency.

STEP EIGHT

"I set a scary life-changing goal."

When I first crawled out from the dark glowing embers of the smoldering fast-food wrappers and charred glass of whiskey bottles that were my past, I was hit by two realities that were not previously obvious. One, I had never felt better, freer, and more scared. Two, now that I had stopped poisoning my body with negative thoughts and actions, I seemed to have plenty of time to rebuild the collapsing edifice that was my life. It was from that vacuum I built my *current* life.

Now… it's your time. The universe has conspired to put you at this crossroads, and you are going to need a big, gnarly, and emotionally compelling goal to get this brand new plane off the runway and into flight. So, your task for step eight is choosing a goal. My guess is you already have one. My instinct tells me you have something that has been rolling around and knocking down bowling pins in your brain for some time - be silent for a moment and see if that goal finds you.

You have created your Avatar. You know *who* you want to be. Now you can choose *what* you want to be, or maybe more accurately what you want to *do*. Think about what inspires you. How far do you want to fly? Do you want to run a "5k" race? Have you dreamt of running a marathon? Ultra-marathon? Ever wondered what it would feel like to ride your bike across the state? The country? Does the idea of climbing a mountain make you feel alive? What is it that speaks to you? What calls out to your soul as you peruse the Netflix library looking at vicarious adventures? You are a physical being, a warrior in the wait, and now is the time to choose your battleground. Before you list the reasons you *cannot* do this... I need you to know my friend Gabriel Cordell wheelchaired thirty-one-hundred miles across the country after reinventing himself... tell me your excuse again?

As you know, I chose running a marathon as the big impossible goal to inspire *me* to do all the work now lying in front of you. I was three-hundred-twenty pounds at that moment, and I had never run a mile before in my life. Yet, I chose the idea of completing a marathon as the source of all my training, the leverage to change my diet, and the inspiration to keep myself focused on moving away from my old life. But understand that it was not the marathon itself that carried me all the way. The real goal was to become the kind of person that runs marathons. That is a HUGE equivocation. If my only goal were getting that finisher's medal around my neck, there would have been no reason to change my diet radically, to go all-in on my training, and to do the spiritual work needed to be peaceful.

I needed the lure of that *life* to pull me through every temptation and every opportunity to fall backward. The pull of being a new person, a marathon runner, helped me say no to chocolate cake.

It helped me say yes to spinach. It helped me say yes to fueling my body the right way and finding a way to be happy while I was doing it. If running 26.2 miles was my only goal, I would have fumbled through my training, walked and jogged for a few hours on a Sunday, and never would have known there was an absolute beast of an athlete lurking inside.

Before you move onto the ninth step, you need to *have* a clear goal. I am not talking about a "lose thirty pounds" goal. I mean something that will create a photograph to be framed at the end of it. An athletic accomplishment. You won't be doing yourself any favors by setting a goal that's just a piece of low-hanging fruit. You need a scary, emotionally powerful goal. You need to want to be the type of person that can accomplish that goal over and over again. Being the person is the goal - not the event itself.

You will never know how strong you can be until you put yourself in a place where being your strongest is required. Oh, and if your goal doesn't shock your friends - it isn't big enough.

Intention 14

It's time to make a significant shift in the way you are working out. It's time to stop "working out" and to start *training*. That means aligning your big gnarly life-changing goal with your actual workouts - time to get on a real training program. So, for example, if your Avatar is a badass marathon runner, going to the gym and getting on the rowing machine isn't going to suffice. If you have pictured the "new you" as a mountain climber, the step mill is a better choice than swimming laps. Make sense? It's important that you start to live the life that you want - now.

In your mind, I want you to be an Olympic athlete. You are training to win the New York City Marathon. You are summiting Everest. When I was three-hundred-twenty pounds and stepping on the treadmill for the very first time, people would have thought I was nuts if they could hear my thoughts. I was acting as if I was a great athlete. Even though I could scarcely run more than fifteen seconds at a time before I needed to take a walk break, that didn't interfere with the reason I was there - to be that marathoner I pictured as my Avatar. Before you scoff at that, never underestimate the power of crazy. The son-of-a-bitch not willing to believe in impossible is the person that changes the world.

I don't know if you have the resources to hire a coach, join a fancy gym, or take lessons for the skills required to accomplish your goal, but if you do - spend the dough. It's worth it. But if you are like I was (the ink on my bankruptcy not even dry when I started my journey), you are going to have to get crafty. There is a ton of free information online. Join Facebook groups, find local training groups for your chosen activity, ask questions, and become a student. There are free groups for just about any sport I've ever heard of. Of course, YouTube can keep you motivated and learning for hours on end. Do what you have to do - but make sure you are developing a clear path to your goal.

If, however, you are already training, or active in a sport, feel free to keep doing your own thing. But you are not exempt from making a life-changing goal. You cannot make this change by running your fourth marathon, but you can by running one-hundred miles - feel me? I suspect there are also aspects of your current training that you have been actively trying to change or implement. Maybe you're a runner who knows you'd be better if you started doing strength training. Or maybe your lack of flexibility has been planting the seed of you trying yoga - if so, do it! Or, if you have been content to be a back of the pack runner, maybe you should make that Avatar a little faster…

MEDITATION

Think about your goal. Live the goal out long-term. Visualize every step it will take to go from where you are now to the finish. Do not rush this. See how deep you can go. Picture the people that you will meet along the way. Picture yourself rising to the challenge, overcoming the obstacles and persevering. Do this again and again… make this a habit and bring it into your workouts as well.

David Clark

ACTION
Train in your chosen sport for at least sixty minutes four to five times a week. Become a student of the sport and give yourself to it completely.

NUTRITIONAL INSPIRATION
Kick-Ass Vegan Pizza - This is technically healthy eating; it will fuel your body and is amazingly delicious too. But we are skating on thin ice with some processed food items, so make sure this is something you indulge in only on occasion or perhaps when you have a big training day ahead of you. I typically use a pre-made crust from the grocery store (try the cauliflower crust). Spread marinara sauce over crust. Put green peppers, mushrooms, spinach, artichoke hearts, and broccoli on top of crust and sauce. Then spread Daiya brand vegan, soy-free, gluten-free cheese over the toppings. Bake per instructions on the crust. Enjoy!

STEP NINE

"I started engaging only in actions that made my new life real."

Today marks the start of a new era, and with it a new way of navigating through daily life that uses your Avatar as the GPS beacon. Obviously, you still have the same mechanics of everyday life: you have to go to work, you are still a mom, dad, brother, or sister. You are still going to be doing many of the same things you've always done, but it should feel like there has been a huge change within you. There should be a feeling that although much of your life remains unchanged, you just see it through new eyes. New spiritual software should be running your computer, now shifting what motivates you and how you choose to spend your thought energy.

Who you have chosen to be is now by default who you are. But you aren't there yet… You are close. You are balancing on the edge of a mountain top. Fall to your left, and you go right back to where you were before you started this program. But fall to the right, and all this becomes real. So, the question is, what will tilt you to the right? Simple - you must now start to follow through with massive and determined action. Your actions following your intentions are the difference between making a wish and making a certainty.

Create a list of the types of actions and behaviors that the "new you" would do. Do you have

David Clark

a role model? If your Avatar was your roommate, what would his or her day look like? Get as real and detailed as you can. It is not enough to just think about this while driving to work; you need to breathe life into this sculpture. You need to hammer on the swirling pictures in your mind until they become hardened like a piece of steel becoming a sword.

This will also help to destroy any remaining pictures of your old practices. In other words, you will use your new set of daily actions to override the past destructive practices. If you used to eat a large, terrible meal before bed, create a new practice such as attaching tremendous value in being the type of person that would never dream of such behavior and that you are a warrior that meditates every night on an empty stomach. Figure out what works for you but make the new associations fun. Envision empowering and bright habits. Remember, these are not terrible tasks that need to be done. Picture yourself waking up earlier, going to the gym, ordering healthy foods, taking pride in how you look, reading books that expand your new life. Make this new identity so attractive and desirable that you *want* to live there.

This is where your meditation practice is going to act like jet fuel for you. To make this new life real, you need a constant connection to your goal. The habits you are creating are an exercise to establish a clear picture in your head of the life you want to live. But once that picture is created, you will need to be mindful of it. You will need to touch it constantly when the lure of junk food comes back.

You will need to be able to feel the "new you" when your mind tells you that working out isn't as rewarding as sleeping for another hour in the morning.

But the good news is this is a temporary tug-of-war. You won't always be in conflict like this. This period of time where you begin to engage these new behaviors is a ritualistic killing of the old you while at the same time, the "new you" learns to breathe. This is where the war for a new life is lost or won. Everyone can change. We all have the ability; the only reason people fail is that they don't stay long enough for the miracle to happen. Here is the final key to winning the tug of war… don't do anything that stands in direct conflict with the goal. Focus all your thoughts and actions on creating this "new you." Burn the bridge behind you and leave no room for retreat.

You are no longer a slave to food. You no longer plan your days, nights, holidays, and rewards based on food. Don't get me wrong; I love to eat. But there is an unmeasurable distance between enjoying a delicious and healthy meal and looking to food for pleasure. Ever met someone caught in a terrible relationship? Ever used the words, "They are in love with being in love" to describe this person (or yourself)? Well, that is the relationship many of us have with food. It's not even food we love, it's being in love with food that we love.

I used to love the way it *felt* to eat, more than I loved what I was eating. I was totally preoccupied with food commercials and memes about food. As addicts, we spend so much energy looking forward to using our drug that there is literally no chance we wouldn't overindulge when the opportunity finally came. The feeling the food gave you was the payoff. It was the "make-up sex." But the relationship itself was damaging you. It was a false high. A roller coaster of devolution that would have eventually killed you. When you learn to see the difference between enjoyment and obsession, you have made a life-altering shift in awareness.

You are also done with giving up on yourself. That is an ugly little habit you picked up somewhere along the way, and we are going to bury that son-of-a-bitch in the backyard. This is your "Rocky" moment. You are getting into the ring to see if you can go the distance. This is the time when you need to allocate every resource you have. Rise to the call and empty the tank. If you do that - it will be enough.

Finally, resist the urge to think of the "new you" as something you will accomplish in the future. You are already living the life you want. You are already that person. Who cares if the proof is a little lagging? If you live the life you want now, the things that are a part of that life will all start to chase you.

Intention 15

Sugar. It's the fucking devil, and I need to tell you that to be successful in the long-term, you need to come to grips with exactly what sugar is. Okay, it's actually not the devil. Sugar doesn't reside in Hell, and it's not to going to poke you in the ass with a pitchfork for cheating on your taxes, but it is definitely a drug. If you choose to keep this drug in your life, it is going to be something that you will struggle with in perpetuity. I can go months without sugar very comfortably. When I am sugar-free, the pull of a vegan donut or a scoop of vegan ice cream is very easy to ignore. I see it and think "that would taste good," but the idea of the payoff is less real than the way I know I will feel after I eat it. So, my brain doesn't even try to convince me to consume the poison. From experience, I know that if I partake in that sugary treat, my entire system will go haywire.

In the fifteen years that I have kept the weight off, EVERY time that I brought sugar back into my diet, I ended up on a sugar-binge for some period of time. One small indulgence becomes another the next day, and all of a sudden, I am eating sugar after every meal. Suddenly, I no longer crave the healthy foods I used to look forward to, and my entire nutritional practice breaks down. I feel bloated, depressed, and my training starts to suffer. Eventually, I wake up two weeks or two months later, thinking, "What the hell happened?"

We change when refined sugar hits the blood. The brain gets instantly rewired, and all the previously solid willpower is gone. I won't revisit the entire topic as I spent much time earlier in this book on it but be aware that should you choose to eat sugar after your rehab, you need to push back hard against the cravings. Have a plan for what will happen after you eat sugar. Treat it with the respect it deserves; it does behave exactly like a schedule one narcotic after all. You wouldn't casually drink a half bottle of whiskey right before you jump on a motorcycle - give the impact of sugar the same respect.

Eventually, I ended my abusive love affair with sugar. The difference was amazing. It makes everything else I do as an athlete easier. I recover faster, I don't feel bloated, my mind is clearer, and I am more motivated. Honestly, once I "detox" (meaning two to three weeks without it), I don't want sugar anymore. Natural foods start to taste better, fruit becomes an almost sexual experience, and my body gives me more energy than I know what to do with. Oh, and you don't have to give up your holiday traditions either. If you get creative, you can learn to make amazing sugar-free vegan desserts. Just make sure that refined sugar isn't stalking you from the peanut butter jar or slipping into your coffee creamer when your guard is down.

MEDITATION

It doesn't matter how many times I have tried and failed. I am not the past. This is my moment in time, and I will capitalize on it. I no longer crave sugar and toxic foods. I am powerful. I am determined.

ACTION

Train in your chosen sport for at least sixty minutes four to five times a week. Become a student of the sport and give yourself to it completely.

NUTRITIONAL INSPIRATION

Protein Triple Nut Vegan Pancakes - In a bowl mix 1 cup of almond flour, 1/2 a banana, and 1/2 cup of cashew milk. Pour batter onto a pancake griddle or lightly oiled frying pan. Cook for 2 minutes each side. Serve with peanut butter on top and agave.

Before going on to the final step of rehab, you should have:

- *Created a new identity*
- *Made a list of new empowering behaviors*
- *Set a life-changing goal*
- *Made an effort to reach out to people from your past*
- *Started training for your goal*
- *Created an action plan that fits your Avatar*
- *Taken a hard look at going completely sugar-sober*

David Clark

STEP TEN

"I stand in the light."

By this point in the program, you should feel pretty damn good. You should be lighter, stronger, happier, and very motivated to keep this new momentum flowing. If you're doing an initial read of this book and have not started the steps, you can look forward to feeling this way soon. But assuming you *are* on step ten, you can take great comfort in knowing you have done the heavy lifting. You are in "The Matrix" as I like to say… you are *right now* living the life that you've always wanted, and it's just going to keep getting better. Although you have likely shed many tears, a few pounds, and thousands of F-bombs, take comfort in knowing that getting to this point is by far and away, the hardest part of this journey.

Before you get ready to check the final step off your list, I should warn you - step ten is different than the previous ones. In a real way, you will be taking this step the rest of your life. Step ten is the ever-evolving, living, breathing step that will be your life moving forward. This step holds the key to you staying on this path and seeing all the unimaginable ways that your future may unfold.

You have done something that very few people have the grit to do. You have gazed into the abyss of your soul, you have confronted all your fears, you have worked your body, purged your mind, and fought tirelessly to free yourself. You have healed your body with plant-based foods, and you have repaired your soul with honesty and action. Do not take this lightly. It is part of human nature to dismiss our successes and hold on to our failures, so do not make that mistake here. If you hadn't found this program, you would still be wandering out there, lost at sea. So just like me, you got lucky.

If I hadn't taken the same steps starting on August 5, 2005, I could still be out there: fat, depressed, or likely dead. I know my friends might think that my turnaround was inevitable. That somehow, if I hadn't made the change on that particular day, it would have been within a day or a week or even a year. But I know now that isn't true. If I hadn't made the leap that day, I likely never would have. That's how it works when you are blinded by the bright light of addiction. Something comes in one day to block out the sun, and you see the wreckage of your life, and you change. But without that break… you never see.

You'll never know why the universe set you on this path, but you should be very thankful for it. Now, it's your job to share the message. I'm not saying you have to become a coach or write a book. But you are uniquely qualified to be the inspiration for someone else now. All you need to do for that is to stand in the light. Be open and honest about who you are and what you have learned. Show people that change is real and that they can do it, just like you did. I can tell you from much experience that if you do not stand in the light, if you try to live your new life in private, you will start to walk back into the shadows. From there, you may end up right back where you started.

You see, we stand in the light, not just for others, but for ourselves to be accountable, to have a purpose in our lives, and to keep ourselves honest. We should do everything we do in our lives as if the whole world is watching because I am sure you see now that keeping things bottled up and buried inside is the type of occurrence that creates the Samskaras you worked so hard to heal.

But be careful. We stand in the light to show that change is real, but we do not lift ourselves to be any kind of leaders or evangelists. We aren't on a mission to save the world, that is an ego-based trip that will make you and everyone you try to save miserable. We live our lives vibrantly and openly and always share what we know when appropriate. That is how we stay healthy, balanced, and whole, and we will rarely engage in activities that will harm us when we are centered.

As you work toward and eventually accomplish your ultimate physical goal, I encourage you to stay on this path. Keep pushing yourself to find what you are capable of becoming. Do not rest on your laurels. I suspect you are starting to feel there is a source of strength inside you that you never accessed before, but I promise you that your strength is a hundred times deeper than your wildest estimation, and your courage is inexhaustible. You were flat out wrong about who you are. You were wrong about so much, so don't be wrong now about how far you can go.

It took me fifteen months of training, of changing my entire diet, doing all the spiritual work you have done in this plan, and losing one-hundred-sixty pounds to accomplish my ultimate goal of running a marathon. But I almost made a fatal error at the finish line. I almost jumped right out of one prison and into another. I almost created a new identity for myself that suggested a marathon was the top of the mountain. Yet, sitting here and typing this, I know that running a marathon has become routine for me. It is something I have done every day for a month. I didn't just learn to run long distances, but I learned to be a peaceful warrior, too. I learned to achieve balance and to become a figure in the health and fitness world. That is pretty fucking stupid when you think about it.

Which is my next point. You must make this tenth step about growing as a human, too. The desire to grow as a human, meaning learning to love more, serve others, and to become selfless, are the keys to the kingdom of happiness. So just as you are going to evolve as an athlete, you need to evolve as a spiritual being. That means reading books, branching out into the community, and of course, continuing your meditation practice. All these can be a source of tremendous growth for you.

Intention 16

I'm sure there are people that have hurt you. We have all been on the sending and receiving side of hateful and painful words. In your journal, make a list of the people that have hurt you. The people that knew just the right thing to say to really make you bleed. Then I want you to forgive them. I know it might be hard to see, but this action is about *your* healing and *your* peace of mind, not theirs. The Buddha said, "Holding onto resentment is like drinking poison and expecting the other person to die."

The people that hurt you were fighting their own battle, and you just got in their way. The more hateful and more personal the words they used, the deeper their own pain likely was. You don't have to email them or call them if that will cause you great stress. But at least start by writing next to each egregious act perpetrated upon you a note of forgiveness. Make sure you do this on paper. This is something that requires clarity and the space to breathe. Maybe someday you'll call them directly, and maybe that day will never come. But forgiving people the transgressions they've made to you will help you move on and clear the weeds threatening to destroy the new garden of your life.

MEDITATION

I am not the general manager of the universe. It is not my job to make everyone happy. It is not my job to make sure that everyone is on task. When I anoint myself as the caretaker of the other people's feelings, they suffer, and I suffer. To think that others need me comes from a place of ego, yet to love and serve others without attachment creates joy for all.

ACTION

Train in your chosen sport for at least sixty minutes four to five times a week. Become a student of the sport and give yourself to it completely.

NUTRITIONAL INSPIRATION

Ultra-Power Salad - Place kale, spinach, and arugula in a large bowl. Put in 1/2 a tub (9 oz.) of spicy hummus. Add sliced walnuts, dried cranberries, cherry tomatoes, cubed avocado, and wasabi peas. Mix thoroughly and serve with a slice of sourdough bread.

David Clark

Chapter 10
Eat Shit and Die

"A warrior lives by acting, not by thinking about acting, nor by thinking about what he will think when he has finished acting."
- Carlos Castaneda

Thank you for coming on this long journey with me. You and I are connected forever, kindred spirits who have seen what lies on the other side of the scary mountain of self-destruction. You instinctively know that humans were not designed to sit in the comfort of the village and survive as long as possible. You feel, like me, that we were made to explore and to shake off the protective lure of complacency and to risk it all to feel something new. You have chosen to take that sentiment to heart and challenge your demons to a fight by engaging in my **Radical Rehab**. For that, you have my ultimate respect and my deep affection. As I've said previously, I think the most courageous act a human being can undertake is to be willing to question themselves and to push back against their own comfortable notion of what is possible.

Now, as you continue to stand in the light and share your journey with others, I want to send you away with a little perspective and maybe even something more practical. Relax, I am not giving you any more homework… instead, I am going to leave you the last bits of wisdom I have to offer on this journey of change. I am going to clean out my coaching garage, empty the desk drawers of my life, and give you every tool I can find to enhance your chances of success. Let's be honest - you'll need it.

Whether someone is looking to lose weight, beat addiction, or build a successful business, most people come up short. But I can assure you that is not because the average person does not have the prerequisite strength to create personal change, it is because the average person accepts mediocrity without much of a fight. This is the great illusion of the masses. A sea of limiting beliefs born of the common experience of fear. Most people tend to live their days in limbo, never accomplishing anything great. But it is not because the human race was only gifted a scant percentage of people that are greater than the average. The force that harvests the mediocrity of man is a low expectation - not lack of ability.

If you don't remember anything else in this entire program, remember this… you are an absolute force of nature. If you can summon the audacity to believe in yourself, and if you baptize that belief with massive and committed action, you will become that rare breed of warrior that does what others scoff at. You can lose weight. You can radically change your entire relationship with food, exercise, and health. You can become happy. You can change your body entirely. You can transform yourself into a solid anchor in the shifting chaos of society. If you didn't

David Clark

clue in yet, this program only delivers you from the evil of food addiction as an ancillary benefit. This program is more of a path to happiness than it is recovery - and you don't see many happy addicts.

I have been very fortunate in my life to be one of the few souls that have made a radical personal change and kept it. I have also been very fortunate that as a part of my journey, I have been blessed to meet, consult, coach, and make friends with some of the most amazing people on the planet. From hall of fame athletes to platinum recording artists, CEOs, gurus, and Hollywood icons. I've had the rare gift of learning in an intimate way how these innovators were able to accomplish what most people only dream of. All that I have accumulated as a student, coach, and fellow survivor of addiction is here in the **Radical Rehab** plan for you. You are not taking only from my experience but from the wisdom of multitudes of individuals that have been able to break free from society's limits and prisons.

With this in mind, I can't send you out into the world yet without sharing a few of the more advanced coaching concepts that you would get if I were your personal coach or if you were attending one of my workshops. So here is the icing on the sugar-free cake, as it were. The five most important paradigms of change. Although these ideas are distributed throughout this entire program, I want to isolate them for you now:

What you are willing to see will set you free.

Let go of what you think you know. Do not buy into your own bullshit. Don't sell yourself a bunch of crap that isn't true. If you constantly make excuses for your failures or your unhappiness, you will never get the leverage on yourself to change. You have to be willing to see your pain, see your shortcomings, and know the *truth* of where you are, whatever that is.

When you want to create a "new life," never count your blessings. Don't say, "It could always be worse." Be willing to see the truth of how bad things are if you want to change them. You cannot beat an opponent if you are constantly denying his existence or minimizing his strength. When you fully accept the reality of where you are, then and only then, can you begin to change.

What you choose to believe is what you become.

It's bad enough when we sell ourselves short or convince ourselves that we are incapable of doing great things. But it's an absolute crime against humanity when we let someone else's limiting beliefs affect how *we* live. Never, ever, under any circumstances, take someone else's advice if they tell you that you cannot make your dreams come true.

What others say is about them. When someone tells you, "I tried that - it didn't work," what they are really saying is, "If you succeed at that, I'll

David Clark

feel like a failure." Maybe they quit on themselves when it got hard. Maybe they dropped out when a family member or friend told them they would eventually fail. Or maybe they just didn't want it as bad as you. Whatever the motivation behind someone else's advice, it has nothing to do with you.

I've run the "Badwater 135," a one-hundred-thirty-five-mile race across Death Valley in July with temperatures of at least one-hundred-twenty degrees. I've done the race three times, which makes me a member of a very exclusive group of crazy people that have finished it. To *everyone* in this group, the race is possible. To almost everyone *outside* of this group, it would be a suicide mission to attempt such a ridiculous task.

If you choose to believe that you are incapable of change, you will be. If you think you're too old, too young, or otherwise compromised in your ability, that will become your reality. If you believe your lifestyle, commitments, career, family responsibility, or any other damn thing prevents you from living the life you want - that is the world you will live in forever.

But if you have the audacity to believe in yourself, if you have the unmitigated gall to accept that you were born with the built-in potential to redefine and reinvent yourself in a perpetual cycle, that will be true for you.

So, surround yourself with others that exhibit the beliefs you wish to have. Model yourself after them. Live in the world where radical possibility breathes, and you'll start to see possibility where none previously was. Understand that when you choose to believe in the words or model the actions of another human who has accomplished what you want, you are not assuming their identity. You are allowing the reality of the universe to live in yours.

Tomorrow will steal your life.

Never let a lucid moment go to waste. It takes a long, slow ramp-up of random occurrences, coincidences, and consequences to become a clear call to action. Millions of internal stimuli in the form of fleeting thoughts and random emotions have fought their way to your conscious mind, bringing you to a focal point. So, take the appearance of this newly formed motivation, and the reading of this book as confirmation that you need to act. The inspiration to change is righteous, and the timing is right, I promise you.

But act now. Do not put it off, not for a day, an hour, or a minute. I lived in the flux of making a change for over fifteen years. A promise to change tomorrow is worthless. Write that promise on a piece of paper and wipe your ass with it - because that is all it is - toilet paper. That resolution is just a casual wipe in an area that will never produce a lasting change.

Tomorrow means never. I have seen alcoholics promise away tomorrow every day until they die. How many promises have *you* already made yourself? What do they all have in common? That's right, they were meant to pause the conflict. To pass the buck off to the next shift. But you *are* the next shift. Believing change will happen tomorrow is the cancer of opportunity. You might think that tomorrow is a new day, but it is not. What you are thinking and doing today is what your whole life is made of. If you can't do it right now on some level, you never will. Do not let this book gather dust. Do not casually discard the opportunity that is laid out in front of you today. Do not let a single day go by without taking action. Create a change now, or a change will never come.

You are not your history or biology.

You are not your parents, and you are not the things that have happened in your life. You sit here today free of the past. There is no such thing as a person that cannot succeed. There is no such thing as a person born to greatness. We are the net result of what we choose to believe, what we choose to see, and how we act.

You have cleared the skeletons in your closets, and you have cleaned the grime from your fridge. Even if you don't fully buy into the spiritual stuff yet, don't dismiss it. Don't throw it away just because it hasn't found the right place to land inside your brain. Spiritual momentum is like your television. You don't need to understand how it works to use it. Stay on this path with an open mind. Even if you fail to execute this rehab the first time - go back and try again. If that doesn't work, regroup. Figure out what went wrong and do it better. Even if you fail a hundred times, you only have to get it right once.

Einstein's definition of insanity is true, "Trying the same thing over and over and expecting a different result." That *is* insanity. That is why you have to try differently. If you hire an expert to teach you how to play golf and fail miserably, that doesn't mean golf isn't for you. It doesn't necessarily indicate that the instructor is incompetent, either. It means you weren't open to what was there for you. You were obstructing the flow of information. You don't always have to change the process. Sometimes you have to change how you give yourself to the process.

If you don't quit now, you never will.

Once you have completed the steps in this rehab, you have a simple task - don't quit. As obtuse as that sounds, it is literally true - if you don't quit right now, you never will. This is why it is so important to stay in the moment. When we overthink things, and when we start thinking about making change in a day, a week, or a month down the line - that's when we feel overwhelmed and throw in the towel. Think about that for a second. Most people don't quit because of what they are actually experiencing in the moment. They quit because of how hard they think it *will* be.

Life comes down to moments and the seemingly small choices we make. Do I go to the gym? Do I eat healthy today? One cookie won't hurt me, right? But every choice has consequences. This is your ultimate work in this program. If you can make just one good choice followed by another, you'll make it. One new action backed up by a positive feeling, and you'll get there. Do not overthink it. Do not judge your journey; just experience the magic of momentum.

I remember while I was running my first marathon in 2006, it was the culminating goal of my entire transformation from a three-hundred-twenty-pound alcoholic to a one-hundred-sixty-pound sober athlete. I had changed every single thing in my life over the previous fifteen months leading up to that race. As the miles ticked off and the pain set in, I started to feel the panic rise. What if I can't make it? My legs were trashed, my feet were hamburger, and yet my family was still 13.1 miles away as I hit the halfway point. How could I possibly run for another two or three hours? I almost started to cry. Did I come this far just to fail with everyone watching?

As I was fighting off the cramps and the burning rage of my quads, a simple thought landed on me. "If I don't quit right now, I will eventually get there." I realized I didn't have to run thirteen more miles on my hamburger legs. I only had to keep running for that particular moment. From that mile to the next. One step followed by another. If I did that, then quitting would never happen. That simple idea, followed by a commitment to keep moving, carried me all the way to the finish and to an entirely new life.

If I had quit, I would have never known the myriad of possibilities that lay in front of me. The battles, the epic journeys, and the amazing blessings that are in my life today. If I would have quit, I would have gone home thinking, "That was dumb. I'm no runner. What was I thinking?" I would have never known that I would eventually run *literally* for days without stopping. I would win races, write books, inspire millions of people, and learn to be happy, sober, and of service to my fellow man. I am NOT a special case.

So, when you are stumbling and ready to drop out - remember you don't know exactly what you are quitting on yet. It might seem like a routine dismissal, just another program you tried and didn't like. But there is a person somewhere out there in the ether. Your actions today are forging this future you. The one who is happy, fit, and burning alive with passion. A person that just might have the next best-selling self-care book in them. A person that will inspire all those around them to live better, to be better. That person is counting on you, and if you walk away - that person dies.

Those are the five big principals of change. If you embrace them, and if you diligently do the ten steps of the program - you will experience a total rebirth during your **Radical Rehab.** Now, while those ideas are alive and worming their way into the back of your mind, let's quickly review the three pillars of this program, and how it all works in the big picture for you:

1. The kitchen is the heart of your life. If you find yourself faltering, slipping back into old habits, or struggling to stay on the path, revisit your kitchen. Have you kept up the ritual of placing only wholesome food in the heart of your home? Do not make the mistake of assuming this cleaning of your fridge was some sort of window dressing. How you do even the littlest of things in life is how you do everything. You cannot expect to honor your body if you do not honor your fridge - every day.

2. If you find yourself frustrated, angry, unmotivated, or lost, go back to the meditation cushion. What thoughts and attachments have you let into your mind? Did you attach your expectations onto others? Did you place your happiness in someone else's hands? Your mind is just like the fridge. If you put garbage in there, it will rot. It will start to stink, and it will spread throughout your home. Commit to keeping your mind as clean as your fridge. Do not let resentment and Samskaras take root. It is easier to clean your plates as you go than to wait until every plate is dirty before you do the dishes.

3. Are you respecting your goal? Is it an actual goal with a timeline, or did you make a wish without

knowing it? Your mind and spirit will rally behind you when you are committed to something big. You will never feel as alive, focused, and peaceful as you will when all your thoughts, actions, and beliefs are aligned in a singular effort. Only engage in actions that support the life you want!

The sum of these three pillars will bring balance to your life. If you are feeling lost, depressed, or out of sync, look to these areas. I promise you that one will be lagging. But remember that balance itself is not a static state. You will never achieve perfect distribution and sustainable equanimity in these areas. One area will come more naturally than the others, and that will lead to an imbalance of focus - and that's okay. If you continue your meditation practice, you will be aware when one area needs attention, and the act of being mindful of imbalance is the road to becoming whole. I said in my book *Broken Open* that we never actually *achieve* balance, it's the act of seeking it that brings balance itself.

So once again, you are at a crossroads. You chose to purchase this book and read it. Now you must choose if you take it to heart. Before you now lie two potential futures. Do you apply the lessons here in a way that makes sense to you, and summon the strength to move away from your old life? Or do you walk away from this **Radical Rehab** and offer some excuse for noncompliance? "That hippie shit wasn't for me," usually works. For the record, if that's how you feel - fine. I can handle someone rejecting my ideas, but what about *your* ideas? If this program doesn't work for you, what will? What is your plan to get better? To beat this food addiction? To go back to eating like shit? Shitty food, shitty feelings, crawling through life led by the overeating cycle? Always wanting to change, but never willing to give yourself to it completely? I doubt it. That's not who you are anymore.

I don't think you would have made it to this final page if that was ever really you. Some unknown motivator kept you engaged to the end. That unknown something is a gift. It is a miracle. I promise you if you squander that gift, it may never return. I called this book *Eat Shit and Die* but not because you will die if you keep eating the way you do. Obviously, we are all going to die regardless of our eating habits. The death that I am speaking of is the death of your essence. The death of the inspiration to live a purposeful life. You were not born to "eek" through this experience, rewarding yourself with junk. Don't let this moment of clarity die unenacted upon.

There *is* a part of you that cries out in the night, isn't there? I know you've felt it. A part of you that knows you were put on this planet for a purpose. That there is something you are missing. If you're honest for just a second, you'll see that you've known since you were a kid that you have something special to do with your life. You have *always* known deep inside of you, there is greatness. You've always been aware of a voice that screams at you from the silence whenever you sit still. You may have tried to give up on that part of you, but it still fights for the light of day.

That voice is what caused you to buy this book. That is the spiritual energy, the karma signature of your life that through a million coincidences delivered you to this exact moment in time. That voice is the true essence of who you are. It's the universe trying to express itself through you. You should drop to your knees and thank God for that voice because not everyone hears it. Not everyone can tune in and receive the signal. That is why I say that recovery does not exist for those that need it. Recovery is for those brave souls that want it and are willing to earn it.

So, do you finally let that voice sing? Or do you slam the door shut? Do you turn out the lights, put your hands over your ears, and hope the uncomfortable pressure goes away? I will warn you that if you do, the voice may never come back. You'll likely go back to eating shit. Back to letting the world tell you why it's okay to fail and comforting yourself with whatever you can shove in your mouth. If you quit on yourself enough times, you might become lost forever. I've seen it too many times to count, and I've attended too many funerals of young people that died old.

I'm glad you chose this time to stand up and fight. You aren't alone. There are millions of us out there battling with you every day, and we have your back. Together, we are the ones that stand in the light

David Clark

as proof it can be done. We are the ones that did the work, fought the fight, and came out on the other side. We believe in the power in others to change as well.

Don't worry about what the doubters say. Don't worry about what will happen if you fail. So, what if someone sees you meditating, or cleaning out your fridge, or writing in a journal? Who cares if they see you training like an Olympian at the gym late at night, or if they happen to catch a glance of you reading your moral inventory out loud? If your friends think you've gone totally nuts - keep going anyway. Your family might even tell you that no one can change who they really are. Co-workers may caution that you can't keep this up forever. Hell, your own family might even say you've turned into some sort of ten-stepping, vegan, hippie, too. People may even get irrationally angry, or say things quite vicious when they see you doing the very things they haven't been able to do in their own lives.

If some "Facebook peeps unfriend you" or talk shit behind your back, take it as a compliment and mark your calendar. Because the same people that ridicule you now will be the same people that come to you one day and ask you how you did it. The same folks who offer up a whole slew of negative prognostications poorly disguised as humor might send you a text message late at night or corner you in the kitchen at a party. They'll be looking for help. They'll be asking for your advice. Or they might even fall on your shoulder in tears telling you they are at the end of their rope with their own food addiction.

When this glorious moment comes, and you become the proof of change for another lost soul, make sure you stand in the light and fearlessly share the truth of your journey. Take no pleasure in seeing them choke back their tears. Instead, remember where you came from. Stay humble and believe in the power of others. But in the interest of paying it forward, if someone that was previously lighting you up on Twitter, or constantly giving you crap, asks you what your secret is… Be brutally honest, look them square in the eye, and tell them *Eat Shit and Die*.

David Clark

Ten Steps Of Radical Rehab

"I promised myself I was done eating shit and acted on this declaration by unfucking my fridge."

"I'm committed to eating only whole plant-based foods for a minimum of thirty days."

"I completed a five-day healing ritual."

"I faced all my demons with pen and paper in hand."

"I spoke my truth to the universe."

"I burned the bridge to my past and forgave myself for being human."

"I created an entirely new identity."

"I set a scary life-changing goal."

"I started engaging only in actions that made my new life real."

"I stand in the light."

About the Author

David Clark lives just outside of Boulder, Colorado. He is a father of three, an accomplished endurance athlete, a practicing Buddhist and die-hard New York Rangers fan. He is the author of the bestselling books *Out There: A Story of Ultra Recovery*, and *Broken Open: Mountains, Demons, Treadmills And A Search for Nirvana*. David is also the host of the acclaimed WeAreSuperman podcast.

Once a 320-pound alcoholic, David's miraculous transformation has inspired millions. He has been featured on CBS, ABC, ESPN, Runner's World, Men's Health and many other national media outlets. Amongst his many athletic accomplishments, he ran the Boston Marathon four times in one day, 48 hours non-stop on a treadmill, and has completed some of the toughest endurance races on the planet.

Made in the USA
Coppell, TX
11 June 2020

27405763R00135